Mindfulness & Nature-Based Therapeutic Techniques for Children

Creative Activities for Emotion Regulation, Resilience and Connectedness

Cheryl Fisher, PhD, NCC, LCPC, ACS

Published by
PESI Publishing & Media
PESI, Inc.
3839 White Ave
Eau Claire, WI 54703

Editing: Jenessa Jackson, PhD
Layout: Bookmasters & Amy Rubenzer
Cover: Amy Rubenzer
ISBN: 9781683732105

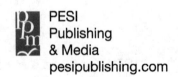

PESI
Publishing
& Media
pesipublishing.com

About the Author

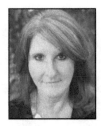 **Cheryl Fisher**, PhD, NCC, LCPC, ACS, is a licensed clinical professional counselor and counselor-educator who presents internationally on the topics of spirituality, nature-based therapies, and overall wellness in mental health. She presents regularly at national conferences in the counseling and mental health industry, including the American Counseling Association, the Association for Creativity in Counseling, and the Maryland Counseling Association. She is a speaker for PESI and regularly presents a seminar on the topic of nature-informed techniques for physical, cognitive, and emotional development in kids.

Dr. Fisher is the program director and assistant professor for Alliant International University California School of Professional Psychology's Online Master of Arts in Clinical Counseling Program. Additionally, she serves as an affiliate faculty member in the counseling and mental health departments for Loyola University Maryland, Fordham University, and Grand Canyon University. She is also a columnist for *Counseling Today*, where she writes a monthly online "Counseling Connoisseur" column.

You can find Dr. Fisher via her online blog (www.cfisherandassociates.com), LinkedIn, Twitter (Dr. Cheryl Fisher @cyfisher), and Facebook.

Dedication

To my nephew, Reed, and all who help save the oceans and turtles and work to make a cleaner, more sustainable world for us and the next generations.

To my grandson, Nicolas, may you inherit a healthier world and grow to be a good steward of the earth.

Table of Contents

Acknowledgements

As with any project, there are many who have contributed to this effort. I want to thank PESI for allowing me to take my passion for nature on the road and sharing workshops with counselors and educators around the country. I am grateful to my editor, Karsyn Morse, for inviting me to create this workbook and believing that I could actually do it!

Editors are amazing people. I recently read "editing is a kind of creative activity where, in a perfect world, an author and an editor find that elusive oneness to understand each other intuitively." My deepest gratitude to my amazing content editor, Jenessa Jackson, who magically crafted a more profound version of my submissions. I am in awe of her speedy response time (I don't believe she sleeps) and her ability to manipulate the text while retaining my voice. Thank you!

My parents, Jane and Shuey Schumaker, contributed to my love for nature by instilling an appreciation of all living creatures. This foundational respect for life creates a sacred space for all creepy crawling, swimming, soaring, and sprouting life with which we co-habitat on this beautiful earth. I am forever grateful for their modeling of good stewardship.

In addition to my parents, I am grateful to my Aunt Lorraine Bailey, whose life has been dedicated to the preservation of all animals, especially birds, bees and butterflies; my *earthing* partner and husband, Steve; my water-sprite, kayak-mate and daughter Steff Linden; and daughter, Heather Lamb, who shares my affinity for the fresh scent of rain; my co-therapists and fur-family members, Max, Lily (deceased) and Elsa who show me daily the gift and complexity of the human-animal connection; and my grandson, Nicolas, who allows me to experience the earth and her creatures in new ways.

Finally, I am forever indebted to Mother Earth and her Creator who entice me to pause from my skim, scan, scroll world and experience the beauty, awe and wonder that surround me.

Introduction

> "Take my hand. We will walk. We will only walk. We will enjoy our walk
> without thinking of arriving anywhere."
>
> — Thich Nhat Hanh

I am not a mindfulness guru or a master gardener. I have not climbed Mount Everest or attended an ashram. I am a licensed clinical professional counselor who has over 20 years of experience working academically and clinically with children and families. I am trained in Mindfulness-Based Stress Reduction, and I have spent the past decade applying the principles clinically, while honing my own practice. I am certified as both a Jungian sandplay and play therapist. I am a certified trauma specialist and have extensive experience in acute care as an abuse and domestic violence specialist in a hospital setting.

I engage in the natural environment through small herb and vegetable gardens, hosting Mason bees and bats, and raising monarchs. I hike, bike, and kayak, and enjoy watching my sunflowers bloom. I am a student of backyard foraging, and nature has become one of my greatest teachers. Additionally, I have a co-therapist, a Goldendoodle named Max, who informs my work with clients and serves to educate me on the importance (and complexity) of biodiverse relationships.

Prior to my clinical work, I was a prekindergarten teacher. I spent hours with my students navigating the woods nearby, creating narratives around the flora and fauna found in the forest. The children and I picked up snails, leaves, rocks, and toads, and discussed their origins and habitats. We jumped in puddles, shuffled along gravel trails, and sunk our toes in the cool muddy banks of the creek. Then, when we returned to school, following a picnic lunch where we discussed recycling and composting, we washed up and climbed onto our hammocks for welcomed naps. This was the children, of course—although I know I was often ready for a bit of shut-eye myself. I found (and continue to find) that spending time outside in all types of weather is good for the mind, body, and spirit.

After 20-plus years as a counselor and educator, I am aware of the challenges in working with children and families, especially my colleagues who work in the school system. There is an increase in children and teens diagnosed with attention deficit hyperactivity disorder (ADHD), conduct disorder, bipolar disorder, and autism spectrum disorder. According to the National Association for Mental Illness (2018), one in five children aged 13–18 are diagnosed with a mental illness. Additionally, 18.6% have used alcohol before the age of 13, 34% have used alcohol or illegal substances in the past 30 days, 13.8% have made a suicide plan, and 8% have attempted suicide (Kann et al., 2014). Often, treatment for children involves a combination of medication and therapeutic intervention, including talk therapy and expressive therapies, such as art, music, dance, and play therapies. However, many of these interventions leave counselors wringing their hands and wishing for more options, as these treatments often attend to only one facet of resiliency rather than treating the entire person.

NATURE-BASED MINDFULNESS: A DIFFERENT APPROACH

The increased demands on children's attention and the additional stressors placed on teachers often results in a climate that is less than optimal for learning. As a result, the need for strategies that promote calm and alert focus and self-regulation are desperately needed. Nature-based mindfulness is one approach that offers a variety of opportunities to promote self-regulation that are afforded by simply engaging in and with the natural elements. In contrast to more traditional interventions, nature-based mindfulness is a whole-brain, whole-body intervention that recruits all the sensory organs through the relational aspects of engaging in nature. Our bodies are naturally attuned to connect biochemically with the natural settings, and nature-based therapy helps bring the body and mind back to its more optimal state. Importantly, it also does so in a fun, accessible, and novel manner that children readily accept.

Have you ever wondered why you feel peaceful and calm after walking along the ocean shore? Or watching the moon and stars from a balcony? Or taking in the deep smell of a pine forest? The earth and its elements—the grass, plants, soil, and water—give off negative ions. Remember your high school chemistry class when you discussed positive and negative ions and chemical exchanges? Well, you can think of the earth as one big battery that is continually replenished by solar energy (radiation), electrical energy (lightning), and thermal energy (molten core of the earth) that produce negative ions. When our body comes into contact with these elements, it responds to the earth by *grounding* our body electrochemically, which naturally prevents chronic inflammation, promotes blood flow to the organs, and increases the neurotransmitters serotonin, oxytocin, endorphins, and dopamine. These changes result in the reduction of the body's stress response, increased energy, improved sleep, and accelerated healing from injuries—in addition to a reduction in anxiety and depression (Ober, Sinatra, & Zucker, 2014). The earth naturally interacts with human (and nonhuman) bodies by promoting a calm, alert state and the overall experience of wellness.

There are many different types of nature-based therapies, including horticulture therapy, which increases serotonin, endorphins, and dopamine through the process of putting our hands in the dirt, planting, and caring for plants. Wilderness therapy is another nature-based approach, which increases neurotransmitters that promote happiness while aiding in vestibular (balance) and kinesthetic (movement) development, which both affect our ability to regulate our emotions. Nature-based therapy can also involve foraging for specific plants or balancing rock formations, which requires practicing focused attention, or mindfulness. It can also include tackling the challenge of navigating the natural elements (e.g., different terrains, temperatures, and climates), which promotes confidence.

Engaging in nature—simply going for a walk, standing by a lake, watching birds, foraging for mushrooms—creates its own therapeutic space. The plants, animals, and natural elements ARE the therapists. **Nature-based mindfulness is a way of using nature and animal interactions in a therapeutic manner that promotes calm, alert states.** In contrast to formal mindfulness practices (which require, well, practice), engaging in nature automatically promotes a mindful presence. By offering our sensory system a variety of novel stimuli to which we can focus our attention in the present moment (e.g., red cardinals against green pine trees, rushing water of the stream, puffy white clouds floating across the blue sky), we are being mindful.

NATURE, WELLNESS, AND DISEASE

I first began researching the role of nature and wellness while examining the therapeutic and healing relationship between humans and animals. As a means of integrating the healing power of animals into my work, I introduced my Goldendoodle, Max, to my clinical practice. I was amazed at how easily my clients of all ages connected with this furry therapist. Max was just Max—a canine who enjoyed human company. My clients would nuzzle Max during session and report feeling "healed" by the furry clinician. However, some of my clinical work did not allow me to bring my canine associate, so I began exploring other venues. This included a betta named Olive, a miniature succulent garden, a tabletop rock garden, and small potted herbs. Still not sure why my clients were responding to these odd and varied interventions, I began to research the role of nature and wellness.

Through my research, I came across the work of Richard Louv, who coined the term *nature-deficit disorder* to describe the increase in physical and emotional difficulties that children are experiencing as a result of spending less time outdoors. In particular, Louv notes that as we moved away from farming communities (where we necessarily interacted with the plants, animals, and natural elements) to more industrial settings (characterized by concrete and isolation from the natural elements), that rates of disease increased. Research has consistently identified a positive relationship between engagement in natural settings and well-being, whereas detachment from nature is related to disease (Berger, 2016; Dietz, 2015; Farmer, 2014; Hanscom, 2016; Louv, 2008).

Yet, in a climate that values curricula that is fast-paced, highly scheduled, and "teaching to the test," providing children time to connect with nature and engage in self-reflection continues to be sacrificed. For example, research by the CDC has found that the average school-age child gets roughly 15–30 minutes of recess per day, often broken into 15-minute increments (Racette et al., 2015). I confirmed this with several teachers and school counselors. One counselor indicated that her school system mandated 45 minutes of outdoor play for children in kindergarten through grade 2, and 30 minutes for those in grades 3 through 12. However, these were also in 15-minute increments. Research suggests that children should be engaged in outdoor play for three to five hours a day!

Growing evidence suggests that this increased alienation from nature is stimulated by modern advancements in technology. As a society, we are characterized by a need to be wired and on our digital devices. Children are on their digital devices for three to eight hours a day, and many schools now require that students to do their classwork and homework on a digital tablet device as well. The more time that children spend indoors glued to technology, the less time they spend outdoors connecting with nature. While this book is not intended to address the information that is available around the role of "blue light" exposure and the increase in myopia in children, parents need to be aware of the real risks of overexposure to digital devices and how to teach and model healthy practices. At the same time, this workbook is not intended to demonize technology. **This book includes the latest research that integrates mindfulness, nature, and technology in therapeutic ways.**

WHAT'S IN THIS BOOK?

Mindfulness & Nature-Based Therapeutic Techniques for Children **examines the whole-body, whole-brain benefits found in nature-based mindfulness activities.** It focuses on the promotion of strengths and less on the diagnosis of pathologies. Further, it offers a multidisciplinary approach to bringing mindfulness, green space, and biodiversity into your clinical or academic setting. It can be of use to clinicians, educators, and caregivers alike. Windows are optional.

This book is comprised of 10 chapters, each of which provides evidence-based, practical guidelines to promote a calm and alert state, creativity, confidence, and connectedness, in addition to facilitating emotional regulation and productivity. Each chapter discusses relevant clinical issues at hand, including anxiety, depression, ADHD, and autism spectrum disorder.

Additionally, each chapter discusses how nature-based mindfulness activities can be useful interventions. While I focus on the preventative and rehabilitative aspects of these tools, techniques, and practices, I also offer an understanding about how to employ mindfulness and nature-based tools with these diagnoses in mind. However, all the tools and activities offered in this workbook can benefit children, regardless of diagnosis. Finally, each chapter provides exercises that are specifically intended to address the relevant therapeutic issue at hand. All information may be reprinted for educational and therapeutic use.

Chapters 1 and 2 introduce the practice of mindfulness and nature-based mindfulness for children, respectively, including activities that promote a calm and alert state. Chapters 3 through 8 examine the benefits of nature-based activities on physical development, sensory regulation, creativity, trauma and resiliency, grief and loss recovery, and the development of empathy and values. Chapter 9 examines the multicultural aspects of nature therapy and mindfulness practices by providing exercises and activities accessible to children of all abilities. Finally, Chapter 10 discusses where to go for additional resources.

The therapeutic aspects of nature-based mindfulness approaches have become a global movement, with research spanning the continents and disciplines. There are workshops, certifications, and entire graduate degrees that provide training about these powerful and accessible therapeutic practices. **It is my hope that this book will serve to ignite passion for the natural world and illuminate the accessible, therapeutic benefits of nature-based mindfulness practices for both children and adults.**

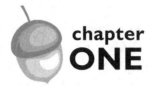

chapter
ONE

Skim, Scan, Scroll Mentality:
It's a Brain Thing

> *"Sometimes you need to sit lonely on the floor in a quiet room in order to hear your own voice and not let it drown in the noise of others."*
>
> — Charlotte Eriksson

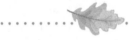

I wake up in the morning to the sound of birds chirping delightfully outside my window. I quietly make my way in the early morning hour to my yoga room where the gentle flow of the tabletop waterfall cascades rhythmically, inviting me to my morning meditation. I inhale deeply, letting the stream of thoughts flowing in my mind pass gracefully in and out of consciousness, and I exhale any tension or tightness my body may be holding as I sit in my deep meditation for a delicious 40 minutes.

BEEP BEEP BEEP! The sound of my alarm wakes me from my dream. I roll out of bed, grab my robe, and fumble to let the dogs out, stubbing my toe along the way. Following a few expletives, I scoop the dog food into the metal bowls, toss them to the floor, and make my way to the hot, steaming shower that must quickly wash away the foggy brain of sleep still lingering. I jump into my clothes, paint on some semblance of a face, and pull up my hair. I grab a glass of juice, a packet of instant oatmeal, and yogurt, which will serve as my breakfast and lunch when I make it to the office. I secure the dogs and (as I exit my house) take a deep breath (holding it for the required four seconds), offer a blessing for the day on the exhale, and haul it to my Jeep because I am now five minutes late for work! (Fisher, 2016)

THE SCIENCE FOR FOCUSED AWARENESS

Although there is a plethora of research promoting the practice of mindfulness and demonstrating its utility, the "skim, scan, scroll" mentality continues to permeate how we go about our daily lives. Children as young as two are being handed tablets, spending hours exposed to blue light and pressing buttons offering instant gratification. Educational forums are capitalizing on this trend by creating clever and colorful educational programs. For example, my 5-year-old grandson, whose educated and loving parents monitor his use, asks for his tablet first thing in the morning. When this grandmother declines his request, he touts with pride, "But it is educational and has animals!" (He knows I love my animals.)

Regardless of the content, there is cause for concern regarding our overuse of technology, especially during the critical physical, cognitive, and emotional developmental stages of childhood. As Carr (2011) describes it, "What the Net seems to be doing is chipping away my capacity for concentration and contemplation. Whether I'm online or not, my mind now expects to take in information the way the Net distributes it: in a swiftly moving stream of particles" (p. 56). We are training ourselves to skim the surface of the sensory input provided, allowing for only a fraction of the material to be processed. Critical thinking and contemplative processes are being jeopardized. Our bodies are being rewired to attend to "hard focus" stimuli (e.g., sirens and artificial lighting) versus the more naturally occurring "soft focus" stimuli (e.g., wind blowing through the trees and sunlight). It's not that technology is inherently bad for children, but chronic, lifelong preoccupation with digital devices is negatively impacting our attention, focus, thought processes, creativity, and productivity (Louv, 2016).

In addition, this "skim, scan, scroll" mentality exists beyond the processing of digital information to how we experience our lives. In particular, it affects how we interact and connect with one another. As adults, we role model this to our children as we skim through morning routines, gulp down breakfasts, throw on clothes, and jump in our cars, only half-listening to each other. We *survive* our day only to drag ourselves home, wolf down something we call dinner (possibly in front of the television), and fall asleep (one hopes). It's almost as if we are living our lives in accordance with the movie *Click* (2006), in which Adam Sandler plays a man who has found that he can adjust the progression of his day by clicking his remote control. He can rewind to times that are enjoyable, fast-forward through tedious activities, and slow down or speed up his life as desired.

Sadly, most of our metaphorical remotes are set on fast-forward. We hurry through our day and rarely stop to pause and experience the moment. In a world that continues to place more and more demands on our resources, this constant state of busyness leaves us vulnerable to both real and perceived threats. We become stuck in a state of hyperarousal. Over time, this chronic hyperarousal can result in sleep disorders, chronic headaches, anxiety, panic, and depression (Kabat-Zinn, 2013). This, in turn, can result in unhealthy coping strategies, self-destructive behaviors, and a propensity for over-reactivity to both our internal and external worlds. In children, this feeling of being out of control and overstimulated can manifest as tantrums and acting-out behaviors. Simply, children are in chronic stress response mode.

I see clients (younger each year) struggling with anxiety, depression, and a host of stress-related disorders. I remember working with a 6-year-old who confided that her first suicide attempt was when she dove upside down off the monkey bars onto the concrete slab on the playground. She had hoped that the fall would have "broken all of [her] bones." Or the middle schooler struggling to maintain straight A's, keep the commitments of her traveling field hockey team, stay abreast of the latest social media angst, and play the self-imposed role of peacekeeper to her divorced parents—all the while cutting because she believes she "deserves" the pain.

My young clients present with ruminations, negative cognitions, body shaming, anxiety related to overscheduling and social status, and parents who are equally stressed. While the manifestation of the stressors may be different, a common contributing culprit is social media and the "skim, scan, scroll" mentality that has permeated our culture. **To get past this mentality and develop a healthier mind-set, we must cultivate a different lifestyle. One that is more attuned to the present moment. One that provides a *balance* between the multiple internal and external distractions and being fully present. In other words, one that is *mindful.***

WHAT IS MINDFULNESS, REALLY?

Mindfulness involves bringing one's focus to the internal and external experience of the present moment, without judgment or attachment. In other words, it involves giving one's full attention to the here-and-now and immersing oneself in the moment. Mindfulness can be cultivated through either formal or informal practices. Formal mindfulness practice involves setting aside a prescribed time to practice mindfulness, such as meditation or martial arts. In contrast, informal mindfulness simply involves bringing a mindful awareness to one's daily activities, such as eating or washing dishes. **Regardless of the nature in which it is practiced, the following seven principles form the foundation of mindfulness (Kabat-Zinn, 2013):**

1. **Non-Judging.** Take a moment right now to just notice the thoughts surfacing in your mind. Then, notice if you are criticizing yourself for these thoughts. "I shouldn't worry about that!" "I don't have time for that!" or "Oh, I don't want to even think about that!" These are all judgments, which reflect the beliefs and biases that inform our thoughts and behaviors. In contrast, when we practice an attitude of non-judgment, we experience our thoughts and behaviors *without critically condemning or acclaiming their presence.* Rather, they simply exist. As we will see in the case study that follows, once Tommy was able to acknowledge his thoughts about horrible things happening to his parents and note them without judgment or response, he was no longer captive to those thoughts. Thoughts are, after all, only thoughts.

2. **Patience.** Patience is the wisdom to know that things will unfold in their own time. However, in a world that promotes the epidemic of busyness, our children are bombarded with messages about multitasking, efficiency, and time management. They learned it from the best: us. To cultivate mindfulness, we must be patient as we relearn how to live with our thoughts and emotions, as well as the sounds, sights, and experiences from which we are so often insulated. This process can be painful and very difficult, as a teen client of mine who was struggling with her sobriety once proclaimed, "I am 16 years old, and I have never allowed myself to feel anger or sadness. It hurts! And all I want to do right now is drink myself numb!"

3. **Beginner's Mind.** A beginner's mind is one characterized by inquisitiveness and wonder, as if seeing everything for the first time. Not needing to be the expert can be so liberating. We want to encourage our children (and ourselves) to experience the world with an open mind and heart. To be curious and with passion. My grandson continues to provide me with opportunities to see the world with excitement and wonder through his 5-year-old eyes. We want to encourage our children to experience the moments of their lives with that same passion and without preconceived notions of how they will experience something. For example, the local news recently called attention to the winter solstice this year, which was to be accompanied by a full moon (known as a cold moon) and a meteor shower. I was extremely excited to enjoy the celestial performance and attempted to recruit others in the celebration. Although the children were just as curious as I was, the adults declined with, "It's just a moon." Mindfulness encourages the awe and wonder of each and every moment as it presents.

4. **Trust.** It is important to learn to honor our own instincts rather than always seeking outside guidance, even if it means making mistakes along the way. Mistakes are teachers, and allowing children the liberty to make mistakes and learn from them is powerful. As Thomas Edison is noted to have said, "I have not failed. I've just found 10,000 ways that won't work." Although we often refer to the "experts" and strive to be like others (e.g.,

a parent, a friend, a celebrity), only we can experience our experiences. Mindfulness promotes an inner silence that allows for the small stillness of our own wisdom to be heard. In addition, the more we practice taking responsibility for our own well-being, the more we are able to begin to trust others.

5. **Non-Striving.** Although I have been known to say that all behavior has a purpose, when we are being mindful, we are not striving for anything in the moment. Rather, we are simply experiencing the moment without any agenda. We are allowing whatever is to be. Whatever that moment brings to us. For example, consider a young girl who is drawing a picture but is becoming increasingly frustrated at not being able to draw the picture she had in mind. The child is overly focused on the end product, instead of the process of drawing. By cultivating an attitude of non-striving, the child can shift her mind-set and just accept wherever the crayons or paintbrush may take her.

6. **Acceptance.** When we practice acceptance, we acknowledge our experiences as they actually are. Instead of attempting to fight against reality, we accept it as it is. For example, if you have a headache, then acceptance involves acknowledging that you have a headache. Acceptance is different from approval, and it does not mean that we condone something or are resigned to it. I find that the notion of acceptance is especially beneficial to trauma survivors because it allows them to acknowledge their stories while understanding that they get to decide how the story informs their larger narrative. In other words, really awful things happen in life (e.g., children may be neglected and abused, parents and guardians may pass away), and it stinks! (That's a clinical term.) There are not platitudes that can make it better, and mindfulness acknowledges this fact by simply understanding that, sometimes, really bad stuff happens. Things are the way they are.

7. **Letting Go.** The final tenet of mindfulness is learning to let go of the thoughts and behaviors that are no longer of benefit to us. How many people do we know who refuse to let go of emotions, thoughts, or relationships that only serve to anchor them in toxicity? For example, I was working with a 13-year-old girl who presented to counseling following episodes of self-injury. She was bitter at her father, who she believed had caused her parents' divorce. She was so anchored in her hurt and anger that she finally disclosed that she cut herself because she wanted to "get back" at her father. She even went so far as to fight feeling better because she didn't want her father to mistakenly think that this meant she had forgiven him. When we identified that cutting was actually hurting her and giving her father way more power over her, she immediately began letting go of the behavior and started working on genuinely releasing the anger, hurt, and obsessive thoughts about her father. While this process can take time, it is empowering to be able to release that which anchors us to pain, suffering, and toxicity.

Learning to be fully present in the here-and-now affords so many other skills that aid in health and wellness. Imagine children who are not critical of themselves or others, who are patient and accepting, who experience life with curiosity and openness, who learn to let go of harmful thoughts, behaviors, and biases, and who ultimately develop internal trust. That is what a practice of mindfulness can offer.

Case Study

TOMMY

Tommy, an 8-year-old boy, presented to therapy with extensive anxiety. He struggled with ruminating thoughts of horrible things happening to his family, and he was petrified to go to sleep because he had nightmares of the same content. He saw visions of his parents dying in car crashes, or his sister suffering through a debilitating illness. While he recognized the irrational nature of his thoughts (even at age 8), he was still consumed by them. Tommy also experienced thoughts of germ warfare, and his hands were red and scaly from his handwashing ritual. When he wasn't washing his hands, he was applying alcohol-based hand sanitizer. In addition, Tommy had been sexually abused by his 15-year-old babysitter. Tommy's sympathetic nervous system was amped at all times.

I have long held the philosophy that successful treatment is twofold in that it must involve symptom management and meaning-making. I always begin with symptom management to give clients the tools needed to address the more difficult process of healing: meaning-making. I also believe that a good night's sleep is imperative to overall life satisfaction. Therefore, I tend to address these concerns first.

Tommy's anxiety, like most, resulted from perceived threats: issues that had not occurred, but might occur! He was overly focused on what might happen in the *future*, as opposed to what was actually going on in the *present*. Therefore, the first step was to bring Tommy's awareness to the present moment, to teach him to acknowledge both his internal and external world as it occurred *in the moment*. To do so, we explored many of the activities found at the end of this chapter, including "Body Scan," "Breath Focus," and "Cloud Spotting." By practicing these mindfulness techniques, Tommy was able to focus on what was happening in the here-and-now, instead of the what-ifs that characterized his intrusive thoughts. These techniques also served to decrease his reactivity and helped promote compassion toward himself. Given that fear of relapse often perpetuates anxiety, obsessions, and compulsions, allowing Tommy to develop compassion toward the possible reemergence of any obsessive and compulsive symptoms incidentally served to reduce the actual risk of relapse.

Additionally, I asked Tommy to objectify his fear and anxiety. I asked him to draw a picture of what his fear looked like, which called attention to his internal world. What color was it? Did it have a texture? What shape was it? Where did it reside in his body? What did he think it was trying to tell him? As he drew pictures of this fear (or anxiety) that accompanied him through this healing process, he learned more about it. He didn't have to be afraid of his internal experiences or spend the energy trying to avoid or repress them. He could recognize them without judgment and call upon them as teachers. It may sound a bit esoteric, especially when working with kids, but I have found that children and even adolescents do well with this practice.

Tommy's commitment, along with parental reminders, enabled him to ease some of his symptoms. However, we had a long way to go to make sense out of his trauma.

Tommy and his parents came weekly, seeking an elixir to heal this young man. With time, the "skim, scan, scroll" of the world was regularly replaced by the scan, breath, and attending skills learned in session. Tommy and his family worked hard each week and committed to the work. In addition to all of their efforts, Tommy's family offered one more strength: their love of nature.

Tommy and his family camped year-round, enjoying the beauty and challenges of the seasons. We had been discussing meditative practices to relieve his mind of ruminating clutter and used the imagery of a river of thoughts flowing through his mind. As each thought came into "view," he was to note the thought without judgment and let it continue to float down the river. One day, he arrived at session with new insight: "I know what you mean now. I was hiking with my parents along a riverbank and noticed how the leaves were floating down the river, just like my thoughts. Every once in a while, a leaf would get stuck on a rock, but after a few minutes, it would just let go and continue to float." He gave me a toothy smile, "That is what you want me to do with my thoughts! Let them continue to float on the river!"

SUMMARY AND EXERCISES

Helping children cultivate an attitude of mindfulness can serve as a buffer against the fast-paced "skim, scan, scroll" mentality of our digital world. In particular, mindfulness practices can teach children to set aside judgment, gain patience, experience a beginner's mind, trust without struggle, accept and let go of that which they can't control, and live in the moment.

The following pages contain handouts and worksheets intended to promote children's understanding of mindfulness. The first handout, **Mindfulness Is a Brain Thing**, provides psychoeducation to help orient children to the negative effects that the "skim, scan, scroll" mentality has on our mental and physical health. It also touches on the benefit of mindfulness in reducing anxiety and promoting a calm, alert state. Depending on the age of the child, this handout can either be given directly to the child or to the parent/caregivers.

The handouts and worksheets that follow contain a variety of activities that introduce children to the primary principles of mindfulness. In contrast to the hard focus that characterizes the busy culture of modern society, these activities promote soft focus and awareness, and cultivate mindfulness practices in an organic manner.

Mindfulness
Is a Brain Thing

Throughout our day, we scan our phones, skim our text messages and emails, and scroll through our pictures on social media to see how much we meet the approval of the invisible audience who *follow us*. To relax, we binge on Netflix or play video games, and we study to the sounds of our streaming playlist. Our brain is constantly filtering the stimuli that is captured through our senses—sight, hearing, smell, touch, taste—trying to make sense of our world. We hurry through the activities and interactions of the day and rarely experience the moment.

As a result, our body and mind become stressed, and the amygdala (the drama center of the brain) becomes overactive. The body perceives that it is being threatened and makes biochemicals (such as cortisol, adrenaline, and norepinephrine) to prepare our body for a reaction of fight, flight, or freeze. The prefrontal cortex (the executive functioning center of the brain) becomes restricted and is limited in its ability to help problem solve.

I don't know about you, but I want the *executives* functioning in my brain, so I want to try to keep my amygdala calm. One of the first things I learned as a student of Jiu Jitsu is to always try to obtain a relaxed (calm amygdala) and alert (active executive functioning) mental state. So how do we do that? One way is to learn to filter the chatter of stimuli and be more *mindful*. That is, to be focused and fully present throughout the day.

According to mindfulness expert, Jon Kabat-Zinn, mindfulness is "the awareness that emerges through paying attention on purpose, in the present moment, and nonjudgmentally to the unfolding of experience moment by moment" (2003, p. 145).

This mind-set requires that we actually press *Pause* when it comes to our busy schedules and, instead, focus on what is directly in front of us. Being mindful *reboots* our system so that we can function better. Bringing focused awareness to our thoughts, behaviors, and experiences in a compassionate way allows us to release that which is unhealthy.

Mindfulness practices have been shown to improve behavior, attention, concentration, and emotional regulation, as well as decrease anxiety, depression, and other maladaptive behaviors.

Mindfulness Exercises

Body Scan

Take a moment and imagine a light just above your head. Imagine this light slowly shining over your head, cheeks, neck, jaw, shoulders, back, chest, stomach, arms, hands, bottom, and legs. Imagine the light shining all the way to the tips of your toes. Do you notice any tension or tightness in your body? Are you hungry? Are you tired? Do you feel warm or cold? Notice how your body feels as you scan the imaginary light over each area. You can take this time to relax any part that feels tense. Where do you hold your tension or stress?

Breath Focus

Have you ever noticed how relaxing it is to take a deep breath? Take a deep breath, breathing in slowly and counting to four in your mind as you inhale. One…two… three…four. Now, hold your full, deep, belly breath and count to four. One…two… three…four. Now, exhale and slowly release that breath. Four…three…two…one. Notice how you feel in your body and how it feels to breathe normally between deep breaths.

Raisins & O's

One of my favorite things to do is to eat! I just love food. However, I often eat without noticing my food. I may be watching TV, reading a book, or (gulp) driving in my car, and I just don't pay attention. Afterward, I often feel hungry and unfulfilled. Try this exercise and see if it changes your experience with your favorite snack. Take a small sample of your favorite snack. I like raisins mixed with Honey Nut O's cereal, or trail mix. Place your snack in front of you. Do not eat it yet! Just look at it. What do you notice about it? What color is it? What shape or size is it? Does it have a smell? (Hopefully a good one!) Pick up a small amount and feel it. What is the texture? Is it smooth or rough? Now, slowly take a tiny bite and just let the snack sit on top of your tongue. Don't chew it yet! Is it sweet or salty? Does it melt on your tongue? Now, *slowly* chew and swallow your snack. What do you notice about the experience of eating your treat mindfully? Is it hard to savor the food? Did you just want to gobble it up?

Cloud Spotting

Go outside, or near a window, and focus on the sky. What color is the sky? Are there clouds? Try to find the clouds. When you find some clouds, watch them move across the sky. Are they moving fast or slowly swirling? What kind of shapes do they make? Are the clouds high in the sky or hanging low? Are they dark (like rain clouds) or light? Spend time just watching the clouds form and disappear in the sky.

Nature Symphony

Go outside, sit by an open window, or listen to a nature app on your phone. Try to identify the different sounds. What do you hear? Are birds chirping? Do you hear wind in the trees? Is there a dog barking? How about car noise? Are there sirens? What sounds does your neighborhood make? Sit for a few minutes and take in the sounds.

Rock Balancing

Balancing rocks is an art, and it takes patience to focus our attention on placing rocks on top of one another. Go outside and find three rocks. They may be the same sizes or different. Sit quietly and try to balance the rocks on top of one another. It is harder than it sounds. Are you up for the challenge?

Moon Walk

Go outside, or near a window, at nighttime. Look up at the sky. What do you see? Can you see the moon? What shape is it? The moon appears to change shapes as it rotates around the earth. What color is it? Do you notice anything else about the moon? Sit quietly and watch the moon move across the sky.

The Elements

Natural elements include water, earth, fire, wood, and air. These elements are everywhere and in everything. Look around you and see how many elements you can identify. Draw a picture in a small journal or take a photo as you find different elements.

Happy Place Imagery

Find a quiet place, either inside or outside, where you feel comfortable. Sit down and take a few deep breaths. You can even practice the "Breath Focus" exercise. As you become comfortable, you may relax your eyes. You may even close them if you would like. Now, imagine that you are at your very happiest place in the whole wide world. Using your imagination, what do you see in your happy place? What do you hear? Do you smell anything? Is there something that you feel on your skin or body? Is there a taste? What are you doing in your happy place?

Spend some time soaking up the scenery in this magical place. After a few minutes, open your eyes and draw a picture of your special place in the space provided. Now that you have created an image of this wonderful place, you can return to it anytime you want—when you feel anxious or sad, or you just want a break.

Group Fun:
Nature Bingo

Nature bingo is a fun group game that can help children cultivate an attitude of mindfulness as they intentionally focus on the different sights and sounds of the outdoors.

For this activity, you will be asking children to go outdoors and find a variety of nature items that correspond to their bingo card. These items can include objects or sounds, such as bird tracks, a spiderweb, or the sound of a bird call.

Whenever someone finds all the items located in a row, they call out "bingo" to let others know they have a winning card. You can download the following free bingo card templates or you can make one yourself. Have children go outside with their friends or family, and see who can get bingo first!

Winter Bingo:
https://www.massaudubon.org/content/download/2744/31934/file/winter_bingo_color.pdf

Spring Bingo:
https://www.massaudubon.org/content/download/2743/31930/file/spring_bingo_color.pdf

Summer Bingo:
https://www.massaudubon.org/content/download/2745/31938/file/SummerBingo.pdf

Fall Bingo:
https://www.massaudubon.org/content/download/2746/31942/file/Fall_Bingo_color.pdf

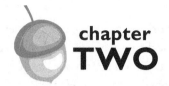

chapter TWO

Nature, Mindfulness, and Cognitive and Emotional Development

> *"At times I feel like I am spread out over the landscape and inside things, and am myself living in every tree, in the splashing of the waves, into the clouds and the animals that come and go, in the procession of the seasons."*
>
> — C. G. Jung

COGNITIVE DEVELOPMENT AND EMOTIONAL REGULATION

Cognitive development is the formation of thinking and problem-solving skills, while emotional development relates to "the emergence of emotional and feeling capacities" (Kahn & Kellert, 2002, p. 120). Importantly, a relationship exists between problem solving and emotional regulation. In particular, cognitive development requires that we have the ability to classify and organize new stimuli as it occurs, while simultaneously managing our emotional responses along the way. For example, if I learn that some trees bear fruit and an apple comes from a tree, I can begin to reason that apple trees exist. However, if I want to go to an apple orchard and pick apples, but I find that the ladder isn't tall enough to reach the juiciest-looking apple, I may become frustrated as I continue to attempt to reach the fruit. When a task such as this becomes more demanding, how do children problem solve and manage their ensuing emotional response of perhaps frustration, impatience, or boredom?

According to Dr. Joleen Fernald, a pediatric speech and language pathologist who specializes in childhood anxiety-based disorders, children as young as 3 months of age should begin to self-regulate their emotions (Hanscom, 2016). However, in this day and age, the school systems are flooded with children (of all ages) who do not know how to effectively regulate their emotional responses. Teachers report that children are becoming more easily frustrated with tasks and experiencing greater emotional disruptions that include tantrums, tears, throwing things, and angry outbursts (Hanscom, 2016). **The challenge for educators and clinicians is to not only provide a stimulating external environment from which children can learn to problem solve, but to also help children cultivate a resilient internal state by which they can manage the variety of emotions that may accompany the challenges.**

The Brain, Cognition, and Emotions

Our ability to engage in higher-level thinking and processing is largely governed by the prefrontal cortex, whereas the limbic system is primarily involved in emotion regulation. Importantly, these two regions of the brain work in a reciprocal manner to inform how we react and respond to situations. In particular, the limbic system functions to interpret the sensory stimuli in a way that assesses for safety first and then allows for the prefrontal cortex to analyze and integrate that information in a higher cognitive format. However, if the limbic system interprets stimuli from the environment as dangerous, then it will override the prefrontal cortex and act in survival mode (Arvay, 2018; Siegel, 2012).

This is great if a real threat occurs; however, without a real threat, this function sabotages the higher-order work of the prefrontal cortex. Therefore, it is important to maintain a calm and alert state to access the prefrontal cortex to its fullest potential. As the following section will describe, engaging in nature is one approach that allows the calming of the limbic system and the full recruitment of the executive functions from the prefrontal cortex. **Calm and alert children are able to better handle challenging situations and problem solve in a more effective manner.**

NATURE AND THE BRAIN-BODY CONNECTION

Nature informs the brain-body connection in several ways, the first of which is through the inhalation and absorption of biochemicals released by plants, trees, water, and soil. In particular, trees and plants produce *terpenes* and other *phytoncides*, which are highest in density in the forest but exist in all areas of green space. The essential oils from plants also possess terpenes. The limbic system decodes and responds to terpenes by releasing neurotransmitters (e.g., serotonin, endorphins) and hormones that are associated with a sense of wellness. The absorption of terpenes also appears to increase the production of the heart-protecting hormone dehydroepiandrosterone (DHEA), which is related to the reduction of depressive symptoms (Avery, 2018). In addition to by-products from the trees, the soil produces a common and harmless bacteria, *Mycobacterium vaccae* (*M. vaccae*), which has been found to enhance cognitive functioning, as well as promote a sense of wellness (O'Brien et al., 2004). Sometimes referred to as "earthing," activities such as gardening, walking barefoot in the sand, sitting in a forest, climbing trees, running down hills, and swimming in the ocean all promote this biochemical exchange (Buzzel & Chalquist, 2009).

Being in nature can also facilitate emotion and cognitive regulation in that it represents "being away." When people are asked to describe their happy place, most people describe some location that is rich in natural elements, such as the beach, mountains, or lakeside. It is thought that this is the case because we tend to "go away" to relax rather than staying in our everyday environment. I am currently examining this "time away" effect through a pilot study that uses nature-informed "time away" stations in the classroom to aid in emotional regulation. These sensory-rich stations include a variety of natural items, such as rocks, a tabletop waterfall, potted herbs, and a small sand garden. When children need to "reboot" and take "time away," they may go and interact with the natural elements for a few minutes and then resume their classwork when ready. In this way, children are learning self-care and self-regulation. Preliminary data appears to be promising.

The cognitive and emotional benefits of nature are also evident through the abundance of varied physical challenges that it offers (see Chapter 3). Natural elements are unpredictable and everchanging. A slow-moving flow of a river in late summer may become rapid in the early spring as the snowbanks melt. Navigating this terrain requires problem solving and the emotional resilience to handle the task at hand. The child may slip and get muddy, and will need to make decisions around how to manage the weather and the terrain. Similarly, when children spend time outdoors building forts or castles with sticks and stones, they become little architects and engineers as they craft their outdoor adventure. **Nature is an endless source of challenges that recruits the brain's cognitive and emotional resources.**

Nature also promotes self-regulation by activating the parasympathetic nervous system, which is responsible for putting the body in a calm and alert state. These calming effects may be particularly salient for children who exhibit difficulties with attention and self-regulation. For example, children with ADHD who regularly play outdoors in green spaces exhibit fewer symptoms than their counterparts who play indoors or on outdoor concrete playgrounds (Taylor & Kuo, 2011). Therefore, the spaces that are used for children's play matter, particularly for those whose capacities for emotional and cognitive processing may be limited.

Finally, one reason that being in nature may help facilitate greater emotional control and focused attention is that it provides optimal sensory experiences that do not overwhelm the brain. The reticular system of the brain processes and integrates sensory information that contributes to our states of arousal and alertness. Environments that utilize colors and sounds not found in nature tend to be interpreted by the brain as "harsh" stimuli and overwhelm the brain, resulting in hyperarousal, restlessness, and difficulty with concentration. Children who are exposed to artificial stimuli in the classroom (e.g., colors, lighting, sounds not found in nature) have been found to exhibit greater arousal and more difficulties with concentration (Fisher, Godwin, & Seltman, 2014). In addition, artificial light (such as that found in digital screens, as well as fluorescent and LED lights) emits a high-energy blue light that places a strain on our visual and neurological system. Nature, on the other hand, provides softer and subtler low-frequency stimuli that is easily processed by the brain and results in a more calming effect.

The sensory experiences provided by nature allow children to interpret the sights, sounds, smells, and tactile experiences in a more integrated manner because engaging with nature is associated with a natural propensity toward *mindfulness*. Nature-based approaches inherently help children cultivate an attitude of mindfulness because the experience of being in nature offers a variety of novel and varied sensory stimuli toward which they can focus their attention and live in the moment. For example, a walk in the forest is filled with stimuli. It may include the crunching sound of leaves underfoot as the wind blows through the trees, causing the golden red leaves to float all around through the air. Birds may be chirping among the tree limbs along with the throaty croak of a bullfrog hidden by the edge of a creek. There is the pungent scent of the wet earth composting the autumn forest debris and moss. If we look closely, we may see the small heads of morel mushrooms popping through the moist soil. All along the path are sights, sounds, and sensations that provide us with a cause to pause, pay attention, and be *mindful* to the surroundings. In this respect, nature offers a free, easy, and organic method to introduce children to mindfulness and promote their ability to self-regulate. **The following section provides a few nature-based examples of how spending time in nature can facilitate the seven principles of mindfulness.**

NATURE AND MINDFULNESS ATTITUDES

Non-Judging

Natural elements are filled with examples of how things exist as they are—how "it is what it is." For example, the natural food chain is neither good nor bad. It exists in the framework of an ecosystem that benefits the entire system. Snakes eat mice that eat seeds left for the birds. This is not good or bad. It just is. Some things in life just *are*, and nature can provide examples of how to sit with the ambivalence of some experiences.

Patience

Nature-based mindfulness provides us with many lessons in patience. A butterfly removed from its cocoon prematurely will not survive. We must wait until it is ready and emerges in its own time. We plant seeds and hope for quick germination. However, timing and readiness is of the utmost importance. As a therapist, I am often amazed at the timing of healing. Nature provides numerous examples of how timing is essential and the benefits of waiting.

Beginner's Mind

Nature is the host of experiences that bring awe and wonder to life. The massive meteor shower on a clear night, the double rainbow following the storm, the sparkle of dripping icicles, or a sunny winter day are miraculous to observe. Children tend to experience life with this enthusiasm, unless it is squelched. For example, I was working with a 15-year-old who was fearful of spending time outside her home following a full-blown panic attack she'd had a few months prior. This resulted in isolation and home schooling. What she missed most was walking in the sand and playing at the beach with her dog. During one session, I suggested that we take my Goldendoodle, Max, for a walk. Without hesitation, she replied, "Okay!"

It wasn't until we were about a block away from my office, nearing the local beach, that my client became aware that she was outside. For a moment, she panicked, looking to me in desperation. I guided her attention to Max and then to the shoreline just a block away. She smiled when she looked at Max and visibly relaxed. She grabbed the leash with conviction, took a deep breath, and forged ahead until we made it to the beach. She plucked off her shoes and proceeded to run with Max, who had been squirming impatiently waiting to play in the sand. The two of them played in the sand, splashing at the water's edge for roughly a half hour. Then we put our shoes back on, brushing off the sand, and walked back to the office. Through this experience, my client was able to experience the walk and the beach initially outside of herself, with Max, until she could reexperience the joy of outdoor play without anxiety.

Trust

Engaging in nature provides us with a multitude of experiences that challenge our physical and cognitive skills. The many and varied aspects of nature help children develop a sense of trust in their abilities to navigate these challenges. However, we live in a society where it is unsafe to be vulnerable, make mistakes, or not get the desired outcome. Well-meaning adults try to protect children from getting injured or experiencing failure, and keep them from stretching their comfort zone. In doing so, children learn that they are fragile and unable to trust their abilities. For example, I was presenting at a conference a few years ago and a well-meaning clinician asked, "What happens if you plant a seed with a client and the most horrible thing happens: It doesn't grow? Won't that be devastating to the client?" However, to trust oneself requires making mistakes and discovering that this is part of the learning process. Life is about the *process*, not *perfection*. So how did I reply to that well-meaning clinician? I smiled and said, "What a great psychoeducational opportunity to talk about disappointment, reevaluation, and tenacity, among many other possible lessons."

Non-Striving

Nature provides us with many opportunities that bring our attention to the experience of "being" rather than doing. For example, my therapy session with the 15-year-old client who feared going outdoors consisted of doing nothing more than having her take my dog for a walk and play on the beach. That was it! No lengthy assessment tool. No worksheet to complete. I simply wanted her to experience *being* back in places that brought her joy. Yes, I know that this was also a desensitization process that allowed her to neurologically supersede her previous experience of panic and replace it with one of happiness and fun. However, that occurred by simply inviting my client to be herself and notice her internal and external world.

Acceptance

Engaging in nature also helps us cultivate an attitude of willingness to experience things as they are without avoidance or denial. Nature teaches us to accept the situations that we encounter without trying to fight against them. For example, interacting with the natural elements means being cold, wet, or hungry at times. These experiences provide a great forum from which children can learn to practice acceptance. "I am cold, wet, and hungry right now. However, I am not always cold, wet, and hungry. In fact, I am usually quite comfortable. What can I learn from being cold, wet, and hungry in this moment?" We tend to spend a lot of time and energy forcing things to be what they are not, and engaging with nature helps get us out of this mentality.

Letting Go

Finally, nature serves as a forum from which we can learn to let go and release whatever is holding us back. The natural cycle of life and the changing of the four seasons provide us with a variety of examples of letting go. Spring turns into summer, and summer fades into autumn, which then withdraws into winter. The day ends and the night begins. Tadpoles morph into frogs, one phase of its amphibian life over as another begins. Birds migrate with the seasons. Nature offers the gentle and organic framework of letting go.

TYPES OF NATURE THERAPY

Spending time in and engaging with nature provides an opportunity for children to learn new coping skills, expand their schema, and regulate their emotions in an organic and creative manner. Given its promising effects, clinicians and educators alike are looking to find ways to utilize nature-based approaches in creative and innovative ways. For example, they are bridging the nature-client connection by bringing students to nature (e.g., outdoor classrooms and therapy sessions) or nature to the students (e.g., using plants, gardens, essential oils, nature views, and sounds in the classroom and therapy session). Although there is no one method to employ nature in therapeutic or academic settings, some other ways to incorporate the researched benefits of engaging in nature include forest bathing, animal-assisted therapy, horticulture therapy, and wilderness therapy. As described by Angela Hanscom (a pediatric occupational therapist and founder of TimberNook, an outdoor education program for children), "whether children are indoors or outdoors, having nature present is a key ingredient to grounding and relaxation."

Forest Bathing

Forest bathing is the process of spending time in the woods and connecting with nature through the senses (Li, 2018). If there is not a forest or nature trail nearby, forest bathing can simply be done wherever there are trees, such as a park or garden. When we spend time among trees, we use all of our senses, which acts as a bridge to promote the resetting of our nervous system. Forest bathing does not simply involve going on a hike or jogging through the woods. Rather, it involves taking in the scenery at a slow and deliberate pace and engaging with all the sensory experiences that the forest provides. Smelling the scent of pine cones, listening to the rustling of leaves, feeling the rough bark of a tree. Although the practice of forest bathing is recently being observed in the United States, Canada, and the United Kingdom, it has been widely used in Japan

(*Shinrin Yoku*), Korea (*sanrimyok*), and China and Taiwan (*senlinyu*) for decades. Many states also have certified forest bathing guides for those who prefer the option of being guided through the experience.

Animal-Assisted Therapy

Animal-assisted therapy (AAT) is an intervention that integrates animals into the therapeutic process, whether in a clinical or school setting. A variety of animals may be employed, such as horses, dogs, cats, and dolphins. Even bettas have provided healing connections with clients. Interactions with animals may be directed by the clinician (asking a child to "teach" a therapy dog the command "sit") or nondirective (observing the child interact with the animal). For example, I have a colleague who does family therapy using horses as her co-therapists. Her first task is to take the family to the barn and instruct them to groom the horse. In doing so, she observes the dynamics of the family play out in the barn. Who takes the lead? How does the family problem solve? What subunits exist? It is quite enlightening.

The efficacy of AAT is, in part, explained by the hormone oxytocin, which is released when we interact with animals. Oxytocin is responsible for the experience of bonding to another, and when a child interacts with an animal, oxytocin is released in both the child and the animal—which promotes a stronger connection. This animal-human connection has particular implications for individuals working with children diagnosed with autism (Buzzel & Chalquist, 2009; Louv, 2016), which we will explore further in Chapter 8 when we examine the development of empathy and altruistic behaviors.

Horticulture Therapy

Horticulture therapy refers to the use of plants and gardens for therapeutic interventions. This process can either involve active involvement (e.g., cultivating and caring for a garden or plant) or passive involvement (e.g., observing the sights and smells of the garden; Growth Point, 1999). Digging in the soil allows for the exposure and absorption of the negative ions and microbes found in soil, which increases serotonin in the body, resulting in an elevated mood (Buzzel & Chalquist, 2009; Louv, 2016) and greater cognitive functioning (Li, 2018).

The use of gardens for therapeutic healing has been shown to be effective in helping numerous populations, including children with autism, ADHD, anxiety, and depression. One of the most recent examples of the power of gardening comes from a high school teacher in the Bronx named Stephen Ritz, who transformed the lives of students considered "lost" in the system by creating a garden (see Chapter 9). The students tended to, harvested, and took home vegetables from the garden. In turn, they started showing up for classes, engaging in the gardening assignments, and improving their academic performance. Through this approach, Ritz afforded an opportunity for these underserved children to reap the benefits of natural settings by simply using a tower garden in the classroom (Ritz, 2017).

Wilderness Therapy

Wilderness therapy focuses on the interaction between and within humans and the outdoors (Jordan, 2015). The experience may last a day up to several weeks. More structured programs may use activities such as kayaking, canoeing, hiking, rope climbing, or mountain climbing. These activities and the various terrains of the outdoors offer opportunities to absorb the rich terpenes and microbes in the air and soil, along with opportunities to engage in complex problem solving. All the senses are recruited as children must physically navigate the terrain, which requires constant attendance to sights, sounds, and sensations. Children may feel a sense of accomplishment as they conquer a fear or achieve a goal, and recognize the power in managing the difficult tasks set before them in the natural environment (e.g., setting up camp, finding and preparing food, managing the weather; Hanscom, 2016; Jordan, 2015; Louv, 2016).

SUMMARY AND EXERCISES

Spending time in and with nature affords many opportunities to engage the parasympathetic nervous system, resulting in a calm and alert state—and a calm and alert brain is better able to self-regulate and problem solve more efficiently. By interacting with the elements, children cultivate a natural attitude of mindfulness that allows them to experience stimuli in a whole sensory manner. Let's face it, I will remember the experience of picking up hermit crabs at the beach more so than reading about them in a book.

The following pages contain a variety of handouts and worksheets intended to promote clients' engagement with the natural elements. The first handout, **Nature-Based Mindfulness**, is psychoeducational and intended to help orient clients (and/or their caregivers) to the benefits that engaging in nature has on our mental and physical health. It also touches on the inherent experience of intention or mindfulness that results from being fully present in nature.

The remaining handouts and worksheets include several activities that promote cognitive development and emotional regulation through the experience of being mindful in nature. These activities promote the absorption of phytoncides and terpenes, as well as the practice of mindfulness. By engaging in these exercises, children can learn to set aside judgment, gain patience, experience a beginner's mind, trust without struggle, practice acceptance, let go of outcomes, and live in the moment. **You can use these exercises with children who have been diagnosed with ADHD, as well as autism spectrum disorder, and in session, as homework, or as prompts for journal entries.**

Client Handout

Nature-Based Mindfulness

> *"Nature itself is the best physician."*
> — Hippocrates

In our busy, overscheduled world, we often forget the importance of being still and quieting the mind. We become overwhelmed and cannot function at our best. We may worry more than usual, have difficulty sleeping, feel irritable or angry, or just feel plain miserable. We may have difficulty remembering things, or our brains just never seem to shut down. To balance our body and mind, it is important to disconnect from the stressors of everyday life and connect with our eco-selves in nature.

Research has shown that spending time outdoors can help us feel calmer, improve concentration, and provide a general sense of wellness. How does it work?

There are natural biochemicals released by plants and trees (called *phytoncides* and *terpenes*), as well as negative ions and microbes found in soil, that benefit our physical and mental health. In particular, these biochemicals have been found to promote an increase in serotonin (the "happiness" neurotransmitter), endorphins (our natural painkiller), oxytocin (the neurotransmitter that helps us bond with one another), and natural killer (NK) cells (cells that improve the immune system).

Additionally, unlike artificial lighting and the harsh sounds of human-made environments, nature provides soft colors and gentle sounds that help to focus our attention and lure us into a calm state, such as the sight of blue bird eggs against a brown nest, red berries on a holly bush, or driftwood moving along a riverbed. In this manner, the earth and its natural inhabitants organically interact with the human body to promote a calm and alert mind, and a peaceful body.

To experience the benefits of nature, you don't have to do anything more than go outside (in any weather), breathe deeply, and experience nature. Notice the sights and sounds. Lay in the grass. Feel the sand between your toes. Smell the flowers. Skip stones across a pond. Make a snow person. Roll in the hay. Simply be in nature. *It is free. It is accessible. It is organic.*

Color Walk

This exercise will help you learn how to focus your attention and be fully present in the moment as you appreciate the variety of colors that nature has to offer. Matching your color cards to things in nature will not only help you focus your attention, but it will also help clear any thoughts that may be keeping you from feeling calm and relaxed.

Preparation

- Squares of color (You can get free paint color palettes and cut them in half to create your cards. You can also create your own color squares.)

Instructions

1. Choose a color from your deck of cards, and hold onto the card as you go for a walk.

2. As you walk, notice how many things you see that are the same or similar color as your card. For example, perhaps you see several deep shades of olive-green moss growing on trees, as well as a dark green lizard running through the grass.

3. Each time you come across a color that matches your card, point it out by saying it out loud or telling it to yourself.

4. Continue to look for things that match this color for 10 minutes. Then stop, select another color card, and search for items that match this second color for another 10 minutes.

5. Depending on how long you walk, you may be able to choose several different color cards. The number of cards you get through does not matter as long as you take the time (10 minutes) to really focus on each color. You can do this exercise as often as you'd like to help develop your attentional skills, but try to do at least one color card every day. The more you practice, the better you will become.

Pebble/Seed Meditation

The following pebble/seed meditation is based on the exercise described in *A Handful of Quiet: Happiness in Four Pebbles* (Hanh, 2012). It is intended to help bring awareness to the moment and quiet your mind. This meditation can be practiced in any location as long as it is quiet. Choose four pebbles or seeds for the exercise, and sit in a comfortable position. Each pebble or seed will represent a different image from nature:

- The first image is a flower that represents being fresh, unique, and beautiful. There is only one you, and you are special just the way you are. Think of this when you are holding the first pebble.
- The second image is a mountain that is solid and strong. You are like a mountain, calm even when challenging things occur in your life. Nothing can move you as you are a strong mountain. Think of this when you are holding the second pebble.
- The third pebble represents an image of water, which embodies stillness. A still lake reflects the images around it. When you are calm, you can see things as they truly are without blaming or being fearful. When you are not calm, you may misunderstand and distort the truth. Think of this as you hold the third pebble.
- The final image is space, which embodies freedom. You need space to move, to be. Without space, you may feel stuck. Just as you need space, people around you need space at times. Think of this as you hold the fourth pebble.

Preparation
- 4 pebbles or seeds

Instructions
One at a time, transfer a pebble or seed from the left palm to the right and repeat out loud:

- Breathing in, I see myself as a flower.
- Breathing out, I feel fresh. Flower, fresh. (*transfer pebble/seed*)
- Breathing in, I see myself as a mountain.
- Breathing out, I feel solid. Mountain, solid. (*transfer pebble/seed*)
- Breathing in, I see myself as still water.
- Breathing out, I reflect things as they are. Water, reflect. (*transfer pebble/seed*)
- Breathing in, I see myself as space.
- Breathing out, I feel free! Space, free. (*transfer pebble/seed*)

Phenology Mandala

This exercise is intended to help you focus your attention on change. Nature is always changing. Day becomes night. Seasons change. Flowers grow, bloom, and die. Bird eggs hatch, and baby birds grow—eventually learning to fly away. Change is everywhere in nature. By observing these changes, you will learn the process of "letting go," which is an important part of being more *mindful*, or fully present, in the moment.

Preparation
- Piece of paper
- Colored pencils and pens

Instructions

1. Draw a large circle on a paper, and then draw four lines (for the seasons in a year) or 12 lines (for the months of the year) extending out from the circle.

2. Look out a window or go for a brief walk. Notice what is happening outside. Is it raining? Is it snowing? Is it sunny and warm? Are there trees and plants? What do they look like? Are they green and blooming or leafless branches? Take notice of any animal activity. Are there birds or squirrels?

3. Each time you do this activity, draw or write whatever you have observed within the corresponding lines in your wheel. Continue to do this exercise on a weekly or monthly basis—whichever you choose—and notice what changes occur in that time. Change happens. It is a part of life. There are cycles and seasons.

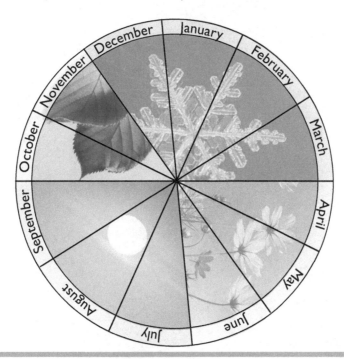

Tabletop Sand Garden

This activity will allow you to quiet your mind while you make patterns in the sand. By methodically arranging the small rocks, shells, and miniature items in your sand garden, you can help calm your mind. Focusing your attention on the movements of the rake or your fingers through the sand and around the rocks, shells, and miniatures enables you to focus your attention and fully experience the present moment.

Preparation
- Tupperware or plastic container with a lid
- Sand
- Small rocks
- Shells
- Miniatures (e.g., miniature rake)

Instructions
1. Place the sand in the container and create a scene with the miniatures. The scene you create is up to you; you are only limited by your imagination.

2. Use the rake to smooth out the sand or make patterns. Allow your mind to relax and notice how you feel after a few minutes of creating designs in your sand garden.

Magic Object
(Transitional Object)

A transitional object is something that is made to represent something else. In this case, you are creating a memory of a place and time when you were happy and relaxed. This exercise will help you imprint that memory of a happy place on a small item that you can carry around with you as a reminder. Whenever you are having a difficult time, you can pull out your object and focus your attention on the happy memory that it represents to feel calm, peaceful, and relaxed.

Preparation

- Small nature items that can be carried in a pocket (e.g., shells, stones, sea glass)

Instructions

1. Choose an item and hold it in your hands (cupping your hands around the item).

2. Close your eyes, and while holding your item, describe your happy place in great detail. You can use the special place you created in the "Happy Place Imagery" on page 10 as a guide.

3. Imagine your happy place transferring from your mind to your hand and being safely placed on your object.

4. Now you can carry and call upon your happy place whenever you want.

One-Minute Challenge

For this exercise, you will practice engaging your senses while being outside in nature. Doing so will help you practice focusing your attention, and it will allow you to quiet your mind and be in the moment. Go outside for one minute, and just sit. Then, answer the following questions.

What do you see?

_____

_____

_____

What do you hear?

_____

_____

_____

What do you smell?

_____

_____

_____

What do you feel?

_____

_____

_____

If I Were a Tree…

Imagine that you are a tree.

- What kind of tree would you be?
- Would you be a little sapling or an old tree that has lived a long time?
- Do you have fruit on your tree?
- Flowers?
- How do animals live with or around you?
- Do you have sap or nuts?
- Do you have deep roots or shallow roots?
- What do you like most about being this tree?
- What do you like least about being this tree?

Draw a picture of your tree in the space provided.

Nature-Informed "Time Away" Station

Research indicates that connecting with nature (even by looking out a window) promotes a calm and alert state. One way to bring this experience indoors is to integrate "time away" stations into the classroom or at home. These stations help children learn how to regulate their emotions by teaching them to spend some "time away" and reboot whenever they need a break from the stressors at hand.

Create a "time away" space where you want children to emotionally regroup. If you have an area by a window that overlooks a natural environment (e.g., garden, trees), that is great. If you don't have a window area, then you may use a digital device that plays a moving picture of the outdoors (e.g., a flowing river, wind blowing through trees). Place a small table in this area that is covered with a variety of sensory items, such as a tabletop waterfall, herb plants, a small sand garden, or cotton balls in jars infused with essential oils.

You can add some seashells, sea glass, or other smooth rocks as well. You may also want to play nature sounds while children are using the station. The goal is to create a nature-informed sensory space that invites children to focus their attention on the sights, smells, and sounds to promote a calm presence. Put out just a few items at a time (perhaps four or five) and routinely alternate the nature items every couple of weeks to allow for a novel and soothing station.

Invite children (one at a time) to experience the "time away" station by placing and setting a timer in the station. When the timer goes off, the child can assess if he or she is ready to return to the classroom or family. You can also use emoji cards to allow the child to indicate how he or she is feeling before returning to the group.

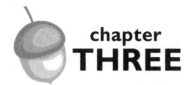

chapter
THREE

Mindfulness and Nature-Based Techniques for Physical Development

> *"The mountains are calling, and I must go!"*
>
> — John Muir

Sally, a 5-year-old kindergarten student, continues to get orange marks on her behavior chart at school, which indicates that she has not been making "good choices" in class. On a typical day, Sally arrives at school at 8:15 a.m. and is escorted to the cafeteria, where she can eat breakfast or just sit and wait quietly until it is time to go to class. Once the bell rings, Sally follows along in a straight line to her classroom, where she is to put her bookbag in her locker and take a seat at her desk. On this particular day, Sally sees Katie and begins talking to her about her new puppy. Both girls get a warning for not going straight to their seats. Sally sits in her seat but feels "itchy in her muscles" and begins to wiggle in her chair. She tries to be quiet, but with each twist and turn her chair squeaks. She gets another warning.

Sally is relieved when it is circle time, as she can now sit on the floor. However, her legs get tired in crisscross applesauce and she needs to stretch them. She stretches right into Adam who yells, "Sally kicked me!" Sally gets another warning. Sally can't wait for recess when she can stretch her body and not worry about hitting anyone. Only, it is 47 degrees outside, and the school policy indicates that it has to be 50 degrees or above to play outside. Today, recess will be indoors, at tables with games or puzzles. Sally picks out a game and accidentally trips and drops the pieces on the floor. She begins to cry. She is overwhelmed with the need to run, jump, and stretch—and now she must sit still for yet another 30 minutes until lunchtime, where she will sit again. She starts throwing the game pieces all over the room. Sally receives her final warning—and gets an orange on her behavior chart before noon.

In our current society, fewer and fewer children are engaging in adequate physical activity. In schools, children are expected to sit in chairs, keep their hands to themselves, and quietly focus on the task at hand for hours. They spend most of their days indoors and are rarely able to participate in nondirected outdoor play. When they get a chance to go outside for recess, children typically participate in 15 minutes of adult-directed activities (e.g., dodgeball, parachute play, etc.) on a concrete structure. In his groundbreaking book, *The Last Child in the Woods*, Richard Louv recounts a conversation that he had with a kindergarten teacher who stated that gym class constituted having children run from the door to the playground fence and back. It doesn't take an expert to know that physical education should involve so much more.

As a result of spending less time in nondirected outdoor play, children are spending more time in front of computers, tablets, and cell phones. The result is a generation of obese, physically unfit children whose motor and sensory skills are underdeveloped. As Angela Hanscom (2016) has described it,

Children are becoming more aggressive and easily frustrated, are having trouble paying attention, are showing more anxiety, and are spending less time in imaginary play…these are due to underdeveloped motor and sensory skills, which leave children underprepared for academics and overwhelmed by daily life and social situations. (p. 3)

Simply put, there is an epidemic of children who would benefit significantly from hours of healthy, regular movement added to their daily schedule, and when children don't get enough outdoor play, the consequences are real.

WHEN CHILDREN DON'T GET ENOUGH OUTDOOR PLAY

As children spend less and less time outdoors, the rates of emotional and physical disorders continue to rise. Children as young as toddlers are being referred at alarming rates to therapy for developmental disabilities and delays. In particular, they are presenting to therapy with lags in basic developmental skills, such as rolling over, crawling, ambulation, and balance—a result of spending too much time sitting immobile (e.g., in baby seats, bouncy chairs, school desks) and not enough time moving their bodies (Hanscom, 2016).

In addition to developmental delays, increasing numbers of children are becoming obese, which is affecting their bodies in a number of ways. According to the CDC, approximately one in five children are obese, and this obesity trend is accompanied by a rise in related diseases among youth, including high cholesterol, hypertension, and type 2 diabetes (Hales, Carroll, Fryar, & Ogden, 2017; Mayer-Davis et al., 2017). Given the prevalence of childhood obesity, children's physical stamina, strength, and endurance is on the decline. They are becoming more winded when walking up stairs and need to take more frequent breaks. They are complaining about being tired with achy limbs. Particularly sobering are the results of a study comparing the physical fitness of children in 1998 versus 2008. In particular, researchers found that children in 2008 could do significantly less sit-ups, had weaker arm and grip strength, and struggled to hold their body weight when dangling from a monkey bar (Campbell, 2011).

I have witnessed these decreases in strength and endurance in the context of my own clinical practice as well. For example, I have a Fit Board tucked away in my office that I pull out occasionally for my younger clients (and myself), who may need to move a bit before settling into a talk session. It is simply a resin board that you can stand on and twist back and forth, or that you can kneel up against and place your hands on to do push-ups. However, I find it interesting that my child and adolescent clients often struggle to maintain balance and take breaks after just a few moments. It is clear that they are not engaging in the necessary physical activity to promote balance, strength, and endurance.

Additionally, we are seeing an increase in disruptive and aggressive behavior, resulting in a staggering rate of children diagnosed with ADHD, oppositional defiant disorder, and conduct disorder. For example, there was a 42% increase in the diagnosis of children with ADHD between 2003 and 2011, with these rates continuing to rise (Visser et al., 2014). Part of the issue is that children need to move! Children are often reprimanded for fidgeting and not sitting still, but the reality is that fidgeting is a symptom of a greater underlying issue: It signifies that children are not getting enough movement (Hanscom, 2016). When children fidget, they are doing so because their bodies are trying to get the movement that they naturally crave and need. As Sally's example illustrates, when this need remains unmet, it can continue to build across time until it manifests in an outburst of behavior that appears disruptive, angry, and intentional.

Given the consequences associated with a lack of outdoor play, some technological companies have attempted to capitalize on the issue by producing applications that incentivize outdoor engagement. For example, Pokémon Go® ignited youth to take to the streets, parks, and community to seek out Pokémon characters that were holographically embedded in the fabric of the outdoors. While this virtual reality game did encourage more kids to get outdoors, their eyes were still focused on hard stimuli—their cell phones and tablets—and not on the flora and fauna growing around them. Therefore, while Pokémon Go did achieve its goal of increasing movement among youth, the research is still inconclusive in terms of how beneficial it was to physical health and well-being. To fully experience nature, you have to ditch your devices before going outside.

BENEFITS OF NONDIRECTED OUTDOOR PLAY

The benefits of engaging in outdoor activities—particularly those characterized by nondirected, imaginative play—on physical development cannot be understated (Hanscom, 2016; Jordan, 2014, 2015; Louv, 2008, 2016). Children need to move, and they need to move in outdoor spaces where they can develop an awareness of their physicality. Importantly, the key term here is nondirected—children need to engage *freely* with the natural environment for optimal development. In contrast to adult-led activities, nondirected activities provide children with the opportunity to trust their own instincts and tune into their bodies as they navigate the earth and all its elements. In addition, spending nondirected time in nature enhances their immune system, strengthens the connection between the body and the self, and provides them with varied physical challenges that build motor skills and self-confidence.

1. **It improves the immune system.** The immune system is instrumental in combatting illness and protecting the body from bacteria, viruses, and tumors. Several studies have found that engaging with the outdoors is one way to improve our body's ability to protect itself against external stressors, as exposure to terpenes increases NK cells, which enhance immune system functioning (Avery, 2018; Li, 2018; Ober, Sinatra, & Zucker, 2014). Simply playing in the dirt, walking along an ocean shore, or strolling through a dense forest offer opportunities for this ionic exchange to occur. Research conducted regarding the benefits of forest bathing has found that spending three days in the forest can have protective effects against cancer by boosting NK cells and other anticancer proteins (Li, 2018).

   Engaging with nature also promotes immune system functioning by activating the parasympathetic nervous system, which helps calm the body. In particular, research has found that engaging in nature serves to lower blood pressure, slow heart rate, and dilate blood vessels by reducing the amount of stress hormones in the body (Li, 2018). Of interest, these results have been duplicated not only in forest settings, but in classrooms where students listen to nature sounds or view pictures of natural elements, such as a flowing river or floating clouds (Avery, 2018). A strong immune system makes for a strong, healthy child—and a healthy child is a happy child.

2. **It strengthens the connection between the body and the self.** Nature provides endless opportunities to develop a conscious and mindful relationship with our body through the sensory feedback that it provides us. When children experience the environment, it is

integrated into their neurological, muscular, and sensory systems. In other words, children learn about their bodies by interacting in the natural world. Snow feels cold, and the body may shiver. Sunshine is warm, and the body may experience tingling as the skin warms.

In addition, nature allows children to experience the wonder of their bodies as they traverse through a newly mowed field of grass, climb the limbs of an old oak tree, hurdle cornstalks, or float along a lazy river on a hot summer's day. As children engage their bodies in the exploration of these challenging experiences, they develop a relationship with their bodies and form a new respect for the beauty and power of their physicality. They learn that the human body is amazing. This new appreciation and understanding of their bodies reflects the development of the "embodied self."

Although digital gaming may give the impression of physical movement as children click their remotes and devices, their bodies do not feel the surge of blood flowing through their veins as they jump over rocks or the pounding of their heart as they race through the forest or the rush of endorphins as they tackle the top mount of a hill. It is only through physically engaging their bodies that children are able to fully experience the embodied self.

In addition, when children develop a positive connection with their bodies, they are less susceptible to the toxicity of the distorted media messages around beauty, strength, power, and identity. For example, I volunteered at a weekend camp for children with disabilities. The volunteers were paired with a child and spent the entire weekend as his or her nature buddy. My buddy was a 10-year-old boy who lived with cerebral palsy. While his muscles were contracted and his body was wheelchair-bound, his spirit was fearless. With some accommodations, my buddy went swimming in the creek, hiked the trail, and plowed through the fields chasing butterflies. At night, he sat around the bonfire with his friends roasting marshmallows, recounting the adventures of the day, and gazing at the stars. My buddy's relationship with his body was one of awe, wonder, and reverence. He truly knew the meaning of living his embodied self.

3. **The physical challenges that nature offers build motor skills and enhance self-confidence.** Being in the outdoors engages the body in a variety of ways that results in strong motor skills and an increased sense of self-confidence. According to Kahn and Kellert (2002), outdoor activities allow children to "explore, interact, recognize problems, attempt solutions, make mistakes, and generate more adequate solutions" (p. 111). For example, negotiating inclining hills or slippery declines, catching and releasing tadpoles or crickets, and chasing butterflies all create opportunities for skill building in a variety of areas, including large and fine motor skills, balance, and hand-eye coordination. As children grow and master these skills, a sense of self-confidence emerges.

In addition, as children navigate the varied and complex terrain that nature offers, they must think through the possible problems and solutions encountered along the way. How can I navigate these rocks to get to my destination? Do I jump across the puddle or craft a walking plank to avoid getting wet? How can I reach that apple? How deep is that water in the creek? If I climb the tree and can't reach the apple, what could I do to accomplish my goal? If I fall in the water, will it be cold?

As children reason through potential solutions, they further enhance their sense of self-efficacy and develop confidence. They learn that they *can* climb the tree and shake the branch upon which the apple is attached. When the branch finally releases the apple and it falls to the ground, they can retrieve it and enjoy the fruits of their labor. (No pun intended!) Most people can remember the challenge of a new skill and the thrill of successful mastery, as the following case study illustrates.

Case Study

KELLY

Kelly, a 13-year-old girl, presented to counseling feeling "stressed" and always tired. She was an exceptional student, the captain of her field hockey travel team, and lead ambassador for her church's youth mission team. Kelly was also in great demand as a babysitter and filled any free time with childcare jobs. In addition to feeling tired all the time, Kelly was plagued with the belief that she was "not good enough." It didn't require a therapist to see that this teen was overstructured, lacking the physical and metaphorical space to explore her "being."

I began every session with a transitional meditation to help quiet the overwhelming chatter of thoughts that accompanied her rigid and overfilled schedule. While it was clear that Kelly harbored automatic thoughts worth exploring, I really wanted to get her out of her head and back into her body. To do so, we would engage in a variety of physical activities, including yoga poses and brief nature walks outside the office. Kelly would rate her anxiety before and after the activities, and she noted how much better she felt when she moved her body with intention. She began to incorporate more outdoor free play with the children she babysat and noticed that not only was she more content, but the children appeared happier and easier to manage after the outings as well.

As Kelly began to see the benefits of engaging in outdoor activity, we spent some time exploring more specific activities that she might like to try. While Kelly was exceptional at field hockey, she had never been hiking or camping. "My mom and dad aren't really 'nature people,'" she confided. "They are more *glampers* who stay in lodges or hotels." However, Kelly was intrigued and wanted to experience a more primitive wilderness. As a homework assignment, she began searching for overnight camps and returned to session with a list of possibilities, including weekend outdoor workshops, as well as residential summer camps. Kelly approached her parents regarding her interest in spending more time in the outdoors, and they enrolled her in a weekend workshop.

Following the workshop, Kelly returned to session giggling with a paper bag she held close to her side as if it were treasure. She gushed about how it had rained the entire time, but she had dressed in her boots and raingear so she could splash in the muddy puddles and dig in the dirt without getting wet or being too uncomfortable. She described digging for roots, picking leaves and flowers, and trying to find dry wood to begin a fire to brew tea from the day's forages. She described using a knife for the first time to whittle and cut pathways through overbrush, and the warmth of sitting around the bonfire with her new friends, chatting away as they sipped the warm brew and nibbled on the roots and berries they had found along the way.

I let her tell her story with detail until we had only a few moments left. Then, I inquired about the small paper bag she had now laid next to her in the chair. "Oh!" she replied, "There was one moment when I just didn't think I could finish the trail. It was filled with boulders and fallen trees, and we had to climb over and under them. Then, we came to a stream and had to walk over slippery rocks to get to the other side. I just knew that

I was going to fall. I took two steps and splash—I slipped right into the cold stream! I was so embarrassed. Everyone was looking at me and there were kids standing behind me waiting to cross. But something happened. First, I was dressed for rain, so my boots kept me dry when I slipped. Second, the kids cheered me on and convinced me to get back on the rocks. Well, it wasn't like I had a choice. I *had* to cross the river to get to the other side. So, I scooped up my pride and got back on the rocks. You know, I fell three more times before I got to the other side. But I did it!"

She was grinning now as she remembered her experience. I smiled and asked, "So what did you learn about yourself in this experience?" She smiled, now reaching in the paper bag, and said, "I learned that I don't need to be perfect to get to the other side. I just need to put one foot in front of the other and keep going. And I can ask for help along the way." She opened her hand, which now revealed a small rock that she had taken as a reminder of her accomplishment. We placed it in her ever-growing "medicine bag" (see handout on page 41) as a keepsake.

How Much Is Enough?

How much outdoor play is considered enough to promote its benefits on physical development? Are 15-minute recesses during school hours meeting the recommended daily requirements? As I have mentioned before, research indicates that children benefit from three to five hours of daily outdoor play, and even younger children (toddler and preschoolers) benefit from five to eight hours! Although the amount of outdoor play can be reduced to four or five hours when children begin school, children should still be offered numerous opportunities for movement breaks throughout the day, in addition to outdoor play (Hanscom, 2016).

Sadly, most education systems are missing the mark and providing substandard substitutes when addressing children's physical needs. Children may receive 15 minutes of recess daily on a concrete slab with an adult-directed activity. While team sports do encourage physical activity and the development of social skills, those types of outdoor activities are not an adequate substitute for unstructured outdoor play. Children need the space to roam, skip, climb, and create forts and communities without adult direction.

NATURE AS A CLASSROOM

In reaction to the outdoor deficits inherent in the traditional educational system, there is a growing movement to bring the concept of early childhood education to the outdoors. All over the world, educators are turning to the concept of nature-based schools to help children reconnect with the great outdoors. In contrast to the typical school system, these "nature preschools" or "forest kindergartens" provide educational forums that are primarily held outdoors. Regardless of the weather, children move, climb, and build in the natural settings most, if not all, of the day. The premise is to have children cohabit with the natural surroundings by engaging in a relationship with their surroundings. Children learn how to navigate a variety of terrain while problem solving the best course. They develop an understanding of temperature. What is cold? Or wet? Children experience the changes of the seasons. They explore animal habitats in the context of unstructured play. Children learn to trust their bodies and problem-solving skills, which builds self-confidence in their physical abilities and in their more primitive instincts.

According to my colleague and nature school director, Teece Nowell, a typical day may begin with an exploration of the woods, where children freely roam, climb, and jump as adults keep a watchful eye. Children are shown how to safely navigate the use of a bonfire so they can heat up biscuits for a snack. The class may forage for berries or edible plants that supplement the biscuits. Following further exploration of the woods, where children identify animals and habitats, they may sit in a field and eat their lunches that have been safely tucked away in their backpacks. Following cleanup, the students resume their exploration and adventures in the natural setting until they are picked up in the afternoon. All the while, teachers are present to provide mentorship and guidance into the children's experiences in a nondirective manner. Classes are limited in size to allow for a small student-adult ratio.

In the past six years, there has been an explosion of these new programs nationwide (Natural Start Alliance, 2017). As of 2017, at least 250 nature preschools and forest kindergartens operate in 43 U.S. states. Many are located in the Pacific Northwest and California, the Upper Midwest, the Mid-Atlantic, and New England. Although these schools are primarily based in the early education sector, there is no reason to indicate that their effectiveness is limited to the preschool years. I was recently contacted by a local principal of an alternative high school who was interested in introducing an outdoor school experience to his students. He described his desire to offer half days to three-quarter days of outdoor education for students who were not experiencing success in the traditional (or even alternative) education forums: "It is as if I need to reprogram them…to remind them of their foundational selves…and help them grow into their best selves. I think an outdoor school experience may provide the needed environment for this work to occur."

For more information about nature-based schools and where they are located, you can visit https://naturalstart.org/nature-preschool.

SUMMARY AND EXERCISES

Engaging in nondirected, outdoor play offers children a variety of opportunities to challenge themselves and achieve mastery over a variety of terrain and conditions, which results in an increased physical health and a sense of agency and self-confidence. For example, Kelly discovered that she did not need to be perfect, and she enjoyed the liberation that she experienced with the unpredictability of engaging in nature. I have employed similar tools with clients whose bodies are challenging. For example, one young client was diagnosed with lupus, which savaged every system in her body. A formerly outgoing and active girl, she withdrew and soon became angry. She no longer had the stamina to go on long hikes or whitewater rafting. She felt confined and betrayed by her body. In turn, we designed an outdoor regimen that allowed her to experience a variety of terrain that was challenging enough for her to experience the sweat of movement, the grit of digging in the dirt, and the concomitant increase in endorphins, serotonin, and NK cells.

The following pages contain a variety of handouts and worksheets intended to increase children's engagement with the natural elements and promote physical development. The first handout, **Benefits of Unstructured Outdoor Play**, is intended to help orient caregivers to the benefits that engaging in nature has on children's physical development. The remaining handouts and worksheets include several activities that encourage children to focus on their bodies and promote active movement in the outdoors. The body is not created to sit all day long in front of a screen. It is intended to move. As counselors and educators, we must work to encourage parents and children to spend more time outdoors and seek out physically challenging situations that promote a strong sense of body and self. Children will find that they are happier and more confident when they move their bodies.

Benefits of Unstructured Outdoor Play

Research indicates that spending time outdoors in nondirective play promotes children's physical development in a variety of ways. In particular, it facilitates a healthy immune system by increasing exposure to phytoncides and negative ions associated with enhanced immune system functioning. Spending time in nature also provides children with a variety of physical challenges that build their motor skills and increase self-confidence.

Further, physically interacting with nature promotes a conscious and mindful connection to the body, including the awareness of the beauty and power of the body. This awareness is referred to as *the embodied self*. Research indicates that when children connect with their bodies in positive ways, they are less susceptible to the toxicity of the distorted media messages around body image. They develop mastery and confidence in their bodies, which, in turn, contributes to overall well-being.

The following are a few ways to capture these benefits of outdoor play and promote strong, happy, and confident kids.

1. Encourage daily outdoor play, regardless of weather.

2. Schedule frequents movement breaks throughout the day.

3. Advocate for outdoor play during recess.

4. Encourage movement prior to going to school. For example, completing a simple chore before heading to school.

5. Save organized sports for middle-school and older children, thus freeing up nondirective play for younger children who benefit from play.

6. Engage in neighborhood outdoor play dates so that your children cultivate a sense of community and engage in the local natural settings.

7. Allow your children to take risks, such as climbing on rocks and digging in the dirt.

8. Allow for more child-led, nonstructured activities.

9. Make outdoor play and daily movement a priority in your family.

The Ecological Body

This activity is a guided meditation that is intended to help you focus attention to your body and how it feels when it is in the outdoors. By practicing this exercise, you can learn to be fully present in your body while in nature, as well as practice learning the skills of acceptance and letting go. You can follow along with the script that has been provided or have someone else read it to you.

Script

Lungs: *Take a deep breath. Begin by pushing the air out of your lungs from the base of your chest. Notice how your body feels inhaling fully and exhaling completely. Our body releases carbon dioxide, and the plants around us release oxygen. It is this interaction between inhalation and exhalation between our lungs and plants that allows us to be alive.*

Heart: *Pay attention to your heart now. Relax and take your attention to the middle of your chest, deep inside. Feel or imagine your heart beating gently, as it has done for your whole life. The first rhythm you were aware of was your mother's heartbeat. The heartbeat is a primal rhythm of nature. It is measured in seconds. Nature is filled with primal rhythm. Our day, measured in hours, is the time it takes for the Earth to rotate on its axis, and a year is the length of time it takes for the Earth to go around the sun. Tides ebb and flow. Seasons change. Just like nature, the human body experiences rhythms.*

Skin: *Notice your skin. Notice your face and hands—any part of your body that feels air. What can your skin tell you right now? Do you feel air? What is the temperature? Is it warm or cool?*

Focus on your skin that is under your clothes. Some cultures wear very little clothing. Imagine what that would be like. Our skin informs us of the world around us, and it provides a barrier for our body. Did you know that skin cells only live for a week? The body recreates skin cells, while letting go of other cells that are not diseased so that the entire system continues to live and grow.

Adapted from McGeeney (2016)

Scuttle Like a Crab

Go outdoors and find a comfortable space where you can practice this exercise. Begin by sitting on the ground, with your legs extended in front of you and your knees bent. Keep your arms behind your back, with your fingers facing your feet. Then, lift your bottom off the ground and try to move sideways like a crab, walking on the ground just using your hands and feet. By scuttling like a crab, you are challenging your body to move in a way that it is not used to, and you are building problem-solving skills as you decide how to move about your surroundings, like a crab. After the exercise, reflect on your experience by answering the following questions.

How did your body feel when you walked like a crab?

_____

_____

_____

How fast could you go?

_____

_____

_____

Was there a part you really liked about walking like a crab?

_____

_____

_____

What part was your least favorite when walking like a crab?

_____

_____

_____

Animal Yoga Poses

Yoga is a wonderful way to bring attention to the breath and the body through intentional movement. In this activity, you will breathe into the position of different animals or insects, and notice how your body feels while doing so.

Find a space, preferably outdoors, where you can spread out. Then, move your body in the various yoga poses illustrated below. You can become a cat as you get down on all fours and arch your back up to the sky. Or you can become a butterfly as you sit on the ground with your feet touching and gently flap your knees up and down, like the wings of a butterfly. Take a few minutes to practice becoming each of the following creatures.

Animal Poses

Turtle	Monkey	Giraffe	Flamingo	Dog

Lion	Butterfly	Snake	Cat	Cow

Which animal pose was your favorite?

_____

Is there a pose that was very hard to do? What made the pose hard? How did your body feel while holding the pose?

_____

_____

_____

Is there a pose that was easy to do? What made the pose easy? How did your body feel while holding the pose?

_____

_____

_____

Nature's Body

Sometimes, we do not realize how amazing our body is. We get distorted images of what represents beauty, strength, and power, and this can negatively impact the connection we have between our physical body and our self. This exercise will help you appreciate and honor your body by allowing you to see how your body fits with the other bodies (animals, insects) of nature.

Preparation

- Large paper (butcher block paper works well)
- Colored pencils, markers, crayons, and/or paint and brushes
- Another person to help you with the first step of the activity

Instructions

1. Find a space outdoors, or near a window, where you can spread out a large piece of paper. Lay down on the paper and have someone trace the outline of your body.

2. Get up and look outside, noticing all the different bodies found in nature. Perhaps you see birds, butterflies, or bullfrogs. Notice how each creature has been formed with a specific function and purpose. For example, birds have wings that allow them to fly. Your body was also created especially for you and the role that you play in the ecosystem.

3. Close your eyes and become aware of your body sensations and how they connect you to the environment. For example, your ears are made to hear the chirping of the birds and the croaking of the frogs. Take a deep breath and notice how your lungs are created to fill with air. Take a moment to appreciate your body and how it helps you every day.

4. On the back of the paper with your body outline, write down or draw all the negative thoughts that you have about your body. Where did those thoughts come from?

5. Flip the paper. Fill the outline with images, symbols, colors, and positive words that relate to that part of your body. For example, if you are grateful for the work of your hands in helping you garden, then you might draw flowers on your hands. If you enjoy certain foods and appreciate the role of your digestive system in helping you eat food, then you might draw a picture of your favorite food in that area of your body.

6. Finally, give your bodyscape a title.

Medicine Bag

A medicine bag is a small bag where you can put objects that remind you of your accomplishments and the lessons you have learned in and from nature. These objects are personal, sacred, and symbolic. For example, when I learned to ski, I collected a very small fragment of a rock (called "shale") that surrounded the ski slopes. When I look at this rock, I remember conquering my fear and taking on the slopes.

To prepare, find a small bag where you can store all of your keepsakes. I like to use burlap, but you can make your bag out of fabric or use a paper bag. Anytime you would like to capture and reflect on your achievements or lessons learned, place an object that symbolizes your accomplishment in the bag.

As you continue your journey, use this bag to carry objects that remind you of your achievements and personal growth. You can bring this bag each week to show your counselor or teacher, and discuss your week of challenges and triumphs.

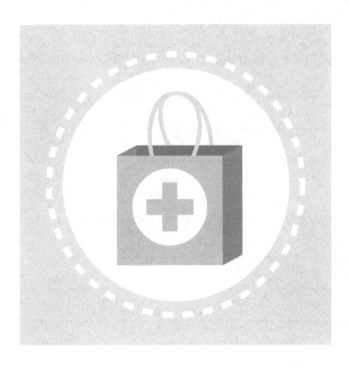

My Body and Movement Reflection

Your body was made to move in a variety of ways. What are some ways that you enjoy moving your body?

_____

_____

_____

What things do you like to do outdoors? Do you like to ride your bike? Or ice-skate or ski? How about walking in the forest?

_____

_____

_____

Are there things that get in the way of doing these activities? Describe them here.

_____

_____

_____

How could you work around the things that get in the way? Who could help you with that?

_____

_____

_____

Now, plan a day where you can do that special activity!

Group Fun:
Imaginary Wilderness Quest

Going on an imaginary wilderness quest is a fun group activity that children can do with their family and friends. Moving through the different landscapes (e.g., jungle, desert, forest, ocean) promotes creative imagery, and it also builds problem-solving skills as children must use their body to navigate through imagined or real obstacles.

When used in classroom settings, this activity can promote healthy movement while reducing fidgeting and restlessness, and it can promote both confidence and team building as children must work together through the imaginary quest. A sample script for this exercise is provided below.

Script

In this activity, you can imagine you are *anywhere*. The jungle, the desert, the forest, or the ocean. Choose a place that you want to visit in your mind and pretend you are there. Travel through the natural setting in a variety of ways that activates your body, as well as your imagination.

First, imagine we are in the forest. What do you see? Let's CLIMB that big tree over there (*imitate climbing*). Oh, I want to SWING on the vine. Let's swing (*pretend to swing*). A bunny just hopped past us. Can you HOP over to the edge of the forest? (*hop a few steps*) What do you see? I see a meadow with lots of bright yellow flowers. Let's RUN through the meadow as fast as we can and SCOOP up handfuls of flowers along the way (*run and pretend to scoop*). Now, let's LAY down in the soft grass and just relax (*lay down on the floor*).

Now, imagine we are at the ocean. What do you hear? The seagulls are swooping down to catch french fries along the boardwalk. Let's pretend we are seagulls and SWOOP down (*imitate swooping down*). Now, let's RUN on the sand (*run*). Ouch! It is hot. Let's JUMP in the ocean water to cool our toes (*pretend to jump in*). Oh, I see a family of dolphins! Let's SWIM to meet them (*imitate swimming*). They are so strong and lovely as they glide through the water. Whoo! I am getting tired. Let's SWIM back to shore and sit on our warm blankets and watch the waves crash on the shore (*imitate swimming*).

Next, imagine that we are moving through the jungle. Do you hear the *caw caw* of native parrots? Stretch high and look far into the trees. The long vines swing from the trees. Oh, and so do the monkeys! Let's pretend we are monkeys SWINGING from the vines (*swing your arms back and forth*). Oh, look! There's a slippery snake slithering from one of the trees. Let's pretend we are big snakes that SLITHER in the jungle (*slither and wiggle on the ground like a snake*). As we slither toward the deep part of the jungle, I see a river. And there are alligators taking a cool bath. Let's CLIMB up a tree and watch the gators play in the river (*imitate climbing*). Whoa! They sure are strong. Do you hear the snapping of their teeth? Yikes! Let's just spend the afternoon sitting in our tree and watching the animals in the jungle, or close our eyes and take a nap.

Finally, imagine that we are in the desert. The sand is so very warm. Do you feel the heat? It is a good thing we brought our canteens filled with cool water. Let's take a SIP of water (*pretend to drink the water*). Ah, that was refreshing. Do you see those prickly cactus plants? One is taller than I am! Let's STRETCH to see if we can reach the top of the plant (*stretch arms up to the sky*). Ouch! It has tiny needles for protection. But wait… What was that creature that quickly ran behind the cactus? Did you see it? It was green, so it was hard to see against the plant, but I know I saw it. It was a lizard! And he is pretty big.

Let's pretend we are lizards and CRAWL along the brown sand (*crawl along the floor*). Pretend that your tail is swooshing behind you as your arms help you crawl on your belly. Gosh, it is really hot, and it's hard to move a lot in the desert during the day. Let's find a watering hole and see if we can find more animals. Oh, over there (*point*)! I see an antelope getting a drink of water. Let's TIPTOE over to the watering hole to watch (*tiptoe across the room*). Isn't it beautiful? What other animals might we see if we stay very still? (*Allow your imagination to create a menagerie of desert dwellers, and enjoy*).

chapter
FOUR

Twirling, Movement, and Nature-Based Tools for Sensory Regulation

> *"I'd like to be a kid again but only because naps were insisted, twirling in circles was acceptable, and the only password I had to remember was open sesame."*
>
> — Adar Burkes

SENSORY INTEGRATION AND BEHAVIOR

Children experience what is happening in their bodies and in the world around them through a variety of sensory organs. The senses that most of us are familiar with are sight, sound, taste, touch, and smell. However, we also have vestibular and kinesthetic systems that help us recognize our movement and spatial awareness with respect to our body and our surroundings. The vestibular system, which is located in the inner ear, aids in our awareness of our body in space and provides sensory feedback with regard to balance. For example, when children navigate the monkey bars at the park, sit upright while going down the slide, or ride their bike through winding terrain, they are engaging their vestibular system. The kinesthetic, or proprioceptive system, has to do with sensory awareness of the position and movement of our body's muscles, tendons, and joints. It allows us to move our body without looking at it. For example, if you ask children to put on their shoes and winter coats, it is kinesthetic awareness that allows them to tie their shoes without looking at the laces, and to zip up their jackets without needing to look at the zippers.

Sensory integration involves the processing of all these stimuli (e.g., sights, sounds, smells, temperatures, balance, gravity) in a way that is functional and not overwhelming. Take a moment right now and think about all the stimuli that you are processing. What is the temperature surrounding your body? Is there a breeze? What are the background sounds? Are there other people talking, a dog barking, a heating or air-conditioning unit buzzing in the background? Do you have music playing or the television on? What visual stimuli is vying for your attention as you try to read this print? Is the light natural or artificial? How does your body feel? Are you sitting in a comfortable chair, slouching on a couch, or laying on a blanket under a tree? Where is your body in space? For you to function, your body must integrate all these stimuli (and more).

However, when children struggle to process what is happening in their bodies and in the world around them, this can result in fidgeting, frustration, falls, aggression, and difficulty with attention (Green & Corson, 2009; Hanscom, 2016). For example, children with an underdeveloped vestibular system may constantly bump into other children or intrude on another's "personal space." Similarly, children who struggle with kinesthetic awareness may complain of lights being too bright, or tags on clothing being "too itchy." They may also avoid activities that are messy. Children with an underdeveloped kinesthetic and vestibular system often experience more trouble with concentration because they are distracted by their own body. Simple tasks such as eating meals, getting dressed, or doing homework may result in frustration and meltdowns (Hanscom, 2016).

TWIRLING AND MOVEMENT

One reason that children may exhibit deficits in the development of these sensory systems is that they are simply not moving enough, and they are not moving in varied ways. Children have an innate understanding that they need to move their bodies in a variety of ways and will do so if not prevented. They will naturally spin or twirl in circles when given the opportunity, and rolling down hills is enticing to the average preschooler. Importantly, it is this very spinning and twirling movement that aids in the development of body awareness and balance. For example, the vestibular system, which is related to balance, is informed by the inner ear. When children twist, turn, and twirl, this activates the cells of the inner ear, which contributes to vestibular development. Therefore, providing children with a variety of opportunities to roll up and down hills, spin on merry-go-rounds, swing on swings, and hang from monkey bars promotes the activation of the vestibular and kinesthetic sensory systems, which contributes to a calm, alert, and happy child.

Historically, playground equipment, such as merry-go-rounds and swing sets, promoted such swinging and spinning movement. However, with reductions in the amount of time allotted for recess and concerns around safety, much of this equipment has been replaced with concrete blacktops and more directive activities, such as dodgeball and parachute. In turn, children are spending significantly less time outdoors crawling, climbing, rolling, spinning, and swinging, and more time indoors with limited movement. When children spend extended periods of time sitting still (e.g., in the classroom, glued to their digital devices), their neck, eye, and sensory systems do not adequately develop. This, in turn, results in poor posture, a disorganized sensory system, and deficits in spatial awareness (e.g., their body's position in space; Hanscom, 2016). We see this often with children who just can't keep their hands to themselves.

Children simply need to move their bodies freely and in varied ways to develop the capacity to integrate and organize stimuli in the brain and body. They need to move throughout their natural environments (spinning, jumping, splashing in mud puddles) to develop kinesthetic awareness (the positioning of the body in space) and engage their vestibular system (necessary for attention, balance, eye control, and posture). These systems cannot develop without movement, which is why in the current digital era, we are seeing more children with underdeveloped sensory systems. Children need to go outside and experience their body in motion—twirling and turning and navigating the terrain—to integrate and organize sensory information.

NATURE AND SENSORY INTEGRATION

There are several reasons that underlie the sensory benefits of nature and explain its role in sensory integration. First, nature is inherently calming. As previously discussed, nature produces organic compounds and negative ions that are absorbed and interact with the body to promote a calm and alert state. Research indicates that children diagnosed with ADHD who are exposed to green spaces (e.g., parks, forests) are more relaxed and focused (Taylor & Kuo, 2011) and, in turn, better able to integrate sensory stimulation.

Second, interacting with nature improves vision. In contrast to the harsh, overstimulating nature of artificial lighting, the visual stimuli associated with nature is gentle on the eyes and promotes eye health. For example, research has found that children who are predisposed to myopia are "three times less likely to need glasses if they spend more than 14 hours a week outdoors" (Ohio State University Center for Clinical and Translational Science, 2014). While theories remain speculative as to why engaging in the outdoors promotes eye health, one theory suggests that during the time of eye growth (ages 5 to 9), outdoor light may help preserve the shape and length of the eye and allow more efficient pupil dilation.

Third, nature promotes children's ability to listen and can assist with facilitating proprioceptive awareness. For example, listening to a bird chirping can help children differentiate their body in space. As they listen to the bird chirp, children must discern how far away they are from the bird. Is it to the left or to the right?

Fourth, nature offers an abundance of tactile experiences that enhances children's sense of touch. Wet puddles, gooey mud slides, slippery reptiles, prickly pine cones, rocky sand, and lumpy pastures are all grist for the mill of sensory integration. So many children are insulated from these wet, cold, windy, hot, muddy, and slimy experiences that they have become tactile resistant. They don't want to wear certain fabrics because they are itchy. They don't like to get their hands dirty or go barefoot. It is for this reason that exposing children to the different tactile experiences associated with nature is so important for sensory integration.

Fifth, the experiences provided by nature enhance children's sense of taste and smell. When children are introduced to fruits off the trees and vegetables off the vine, they are able to experience the crisp flavor of a freshly picked apple or the fragrant scent of citrus from an orange blossom tree.

Finally, the rich and varied settings of nature promote movement and exploration. Grassy knolls, dry deserts, muddy swamps, rough-barked trees, and cool, wet ponds each beckon the child to explore their vastness. Children are natural scientists, curious and adventuresome. If not deterred, many will naturally investigate by running, jumping, climbing, and crawling through their environments.

Simply put, being in nature promotes less sensory overload and exposes children to a variety of tactile stimuli, while increasing vestibular engagement through movement and play. It provides a whole-brain, whole-body exposure to an abundance of natural stimuli and varied terrain. It is in the context of natural settings where sensory integration occurs.

SENSORY DISORGANIZATION, BEHAVIOR, AND MENTAL HEALTH

Given the important role that nature plays in sensory integration, it is not surprising that a lack of outdoor play is associated with an inability to integrate and organize sensory information. When children experience sensory disintegration, they are unable to process the basic information that they receive about their bodies and the world around them. That is, they are unable to filter and organize the feedback they receive through their sense of sight, sound, touch, balance, etc. Their inability to successfully integrate incoming stimuli results in sensory overload, which activates the sympathetic nervous system and puts the body in fight, flight, or freeze mode. It causes their nervous system to react as if it is in danger. When this activation goes on for an extended period of time, children become overwhelmed, which can result in restlessness, an inability to concentrate, agitation, and possibly aggressive behavior.

At its most extreme, difficulties with sensory integration are associated with sensory processing disorder (SPD), which is a complex and often misunderstood disorder that is frequently misdiagnosed. Essentially on a continuum, children with SPD may exhibit a variety of processing challenges, which can involve being hyposensitive, hypersensitive, or sensory seeking.

Children with SPD who are hyposensitive are under-responsive to sensory stimuli. As a result, they often have a high threshold for pain and seem unbothered by injuries or extremes in temperature. They may exhibit poor social skills because they fail to detect sensory input in their environment (e.g., an adult or peer calling their name). Children who are hyposensitive also exhibit poor body awareness, which can lead to difficulties with clumsiness and lack of coordination.

On the other hand, children with SPD can be hypersensitive in that they have a low threshold for sensation and experience sensory stimuli as overwhelming. Because they are easily overstimulated, these children react poorly when they hear sudden, loud noises or are touched unexpectedly. They frequently have aversions to certain textures and sensations (e.g., tags on clothing, the feeling of sand, certain foods). Their fight, flight, or freeze system is on high alert, which can result in behavioral outbursts and aggression toward others in response to perceived threats. These children may also create rigid routines in attempts to avoid or escape stimuli. Often, children who are hypersensitive are described as "anxious, aggressive, distracted or unfocused, or as picky eaters" (Goodman-Scott & Lambert, 2015, p. 275).

Last, children with SPD can be sensory seeking in that they actively seek constant movement to receive sensations from their environment. They are seen constantly running, jumping, chewing, tapping, humming, and squeezing. They may excessively seek out textures and surfaces that provide them with sensory stimulation, and they may touch other people because of difficulties discriminating personal space. Children who are sensory seeking may appear "impulsive, unpredictable, and have inappropriate personal space and are often described as rambunctious, aggressive, or bouncing off the walls" (Goodman-Scott & Lambert, 2015, p. 275).

It is not just SPD that involves sensory processing issues, as children with ADHD can have significant problems with sensory integration as well. For example, in classroom settings, children with ADHD may struggle to filter out the noise of other children whispering nearby, which contributes to difficulties paying attention. Additionally, they may become fidgety and restless, requiring frequent movement. As a result, children with ADHD may leave their seat often and run or climb when inappropriate. Additionally, research indicates that over half of the children diagnosed with ADHD have balance and motor coordination deficits (Faramarzi, Rad, & Abedi, 2016).

Because SPD and ADHD have similar behavior profiles (e.g., excessive activity, impulsivity, sensation seeking, and distractibility; Delaney, 2008), SPD is often misdiagnosed as ADHD. In addition, there are times when the disorders co-occur, as research indicates that 40% of children with ADHD also have SPD (Ahn, Miller, Milberger, & McIntosh, 2004). Although the two disorders have similar manifestations and frequently co-occur, children impacted by ADHD have historically been treated with medication and behavior therapy, whereas children with SPD have received sensory integration treatment often provided by occupational therapists. More recently, research suggests that children affected by both ADHD and SPD can benefit from sensory-focused approaches (Koenig, Huecker, & Kinneally, 2005; Taylor & Kuo, 2011), as the following framework demonstrates.

A Framework for Treating Sensory Disintegration

Occupational therapists Abigail Green and Diane Corson (2009) have identified the relationship between sensory integration and manifested behavior in children, from which they have developed a framework for assessing and treating sensory processing issues, see **Anaylsis of Sensory Behaviors: Planning Worksheet**, page 63. Broadly speaking, their framework involves (1) listing the child's observed problem behaviors (e.g., hitting, biting, inattentive, restless) and identifying the accompanying sensory systems involved (e.g., auditory, tactile, vestibular). The next step is to (2) assess the child's environment for change. For example, a simple modification might include having the child sit by a window for natural light. Following an environmental assessment, there is a (3) development of sensory tasks (longer and mini) that can address the child's sensory issues and promote desired behavior. For example, perhaps the child would benefit from sitting on a balance ball for kinesthetic awareness during circle time (longer sensory task), or from putting on hand lotion for tactile stimulation (mini sensory task).

Finally, a (4) **Sensory Diet Plan** (page 64) is included that can be implemented for use at school, at home, and in clinical sessions. The sensory diet plan is a structured routine for the child that offers large sensory tasks, as well as mini sensory break ideas, at scheduled times. For example, a child who is continuously moving in his or her chair may benefit from doing table activities, like reading and writing, while sitting on a balance ball, and taking mini-movement breaks that include standing and stretching every half hour. You can use this sensory structure routine as part of the child's treatment plan and integrate it into his or her individual educational plan (IEP) in the context of the school setting. As the following case study will illustrate, this framework can effectively address and treat behavioral issues that represent manifestations of underlying sensory issues.

Case Study

KEVIN

Kevin, an 8-year-old boy, presented to my practice after being diagnosed with ADHD, inattentive type. He was described by family and teachers as inattentive, disruptive, argumentative, restless, and difficult, often interrupting others. He became angry and defensive whenever he was confronted about his behavior, and he held the belief that he was a "bad boy" and "nobody likes me." He liked reptiles and toads, and he had a pet lizard. One of his favorite activities also involved crabbing with his uncle.

Kevin lived with his parents in a suburban community, though he attended a private school in the city. Every day during the week, his parents would leave early to drive him (25 miles one way) to school, where he immediately went to his SMART classroom and sat for hours in front of the latest digital technology. The curriculum was rigorous, which only allowed for a 15-minute recess that involved semi-restrictive play on a concrete playground. Kevin and his friends would usually play games on their tablets or phones, which they were allowed to access at recess. After recess, he would return to the classroom for several more hours and then work on his homework during the hour ride home in rush-hour traffic. When he got home, it was time to take care of his lizard, eat dinner, and prepare for the next day. Like many children who have privileged lives of structure and adult-led activities, Kevin was not afforded the luxury of free time and outdoor play.

Using the sensory skills framework developed by Green and Corson (2009), I identified Kevin's behaviors of concern as inattentiveness, restlessness, and disruptive behavior (e.g., fidgets, throws things at other children, interrupts). The sensory systems that were impacted included vestibular (restlessness and inattentiveness) and visual (sensitive to artificial lighting). An assessment revealed that his classroom environment was restrictive, as Kevin was expected to sit in his chair for extended periods of time, where he was exposed to hours of blue light emitted from the SMART board, with limited time for nondirected play or movement. The artificial lighting added to Kevin's overstimulated sensory system.

Some specific sensory tasks were developed to address Kevin's specific needs, which included increasing his movement through spin breaks, sitting on a therapy ball for movement in place, and increasing his access to natural stimuli through a nature-informed sensory room. Finally, a sensory structure routine was put in place allowing Kevin to (1) take mini-movement breaks to stretch and spin, (2) use a therapy ball instead of a regular chair, (3) go to the nature-informed sensory space when he was feeling agitated, (4) use lotion to soothe his body when needed, and (5) wrap himself in a soft blanket for soothing as needed.

In addition to attending to sensory stimuli, Kevin was provided with more outdoor opportunities during the week and weekend. While these opportunities were more limited during the week, Kevin was still instructed to go outside every night for a minimum of 15 to 20 minutes and to draw a picture of what he saw, heard, and experienced. This exercise formed the basis of his journal, which he brought to therapy each week. Additionally, because Kevin's behavior had alienated him from many of his peers, he was allowed to bring his lizard to school so he could teach his classmates about caring for a lizard. Needless to say, Kevin became quite the hero following his show-and-tell. Finally, as a positive reward for his conscious efforts toward change, Kevin was provided with a weekend trip of crabbing and fishing with his beloved uncle.

Of little surprise, Kevin's behavior changed drastically. As a result of providing Kevin with adequate and regular opportunities for movement, along with natural sensory stimulation via outdoor activity, his ability to focus improved, and he was less restless and disruptive. Because of Kevin's success, his teacher even began to implement several of these strategies (e.g., spin breaks, therapy balls, and sensory breaks) into her classroom management system, which allowed all of her students more opportunities for movement and sensory breaks.

SUMMARY AND EXERCISES

Children are sensory-oriented beings, intended to experience their human existence in a holistic manner. They are not intended to sit for hours in artificial lighting with artificial sounds and experience life from a chair in front of a digital screen. Children are wired to take in a variety of stimuli through their sensory systems, including their eyes, ears, hands, feet, and sense of balance. However, if they are restricted in their experiences, their sensory processing systems cannot fully develop, which renders them unable to make sense of what is happening in their bodies and in the world around them. They become overwhelmed as a result of being in a chronic state of sensory overload, causing them to become fidgety, restless, aggressive, and intolerant of varied stimuli.

Being in nature can help children return to a state of sensory integration and organization through the plethora of sensory-rich opportunities that the natural settings provide. When children are outdoors, they have the freedom to run, jump, climb, and explore a variety of terrain, in turn facilitating tactile engagement, kinesthetic awareness, and vestibular engagement.

The following pages provide a variety of fun and creative activities that promote sensory integration by encouraging children's engagement with natural stimuli. The first handout is intended to orient caregivers and educators to the concept of sensory integration and the benefits of nature in helping children process and organize sensory stimuli in a functional manner. The exercises that follow can be of benefit to children who struggle with sensory issues, including those who exhibit symptomology associated with ADHD and SPD, as these activities promote sensory awareness and integration. As Richard Louv notes, "Time in nature is not leisure time; it's an essential investment in our children's health (and also, by the way, in our own)" (2008, p. 120).

Nature and Sensory Integration

Children experience what is happening in their bodies and in the world around them through their senses. This includes the most commonly thought of senses (e.g., sight, sound, smell, taste, touch), as well as the senses associated with the kinesthetic system (awareness of body in space and movement) and vestibular system (balance and movement). Children require some stimulation for these sensory systems to grow and develop in a healthy manner.

However, too much stimulation (such as that from artificial light and sirens) can be overwhelming, while too little stimulation can restrict development. In contrast, the variety of sensory experiences supplied by nature offer the right amount of stimulation to help children develop the ability to process all stimuli (e.g., sights, sounds, smells, temperatures, balance, gravity) in a way that is functional and not overwhelming. The are several reasons that nature has these benefits:

- **Nature is calming.** Viewing nature has a soothing effect. While being outdoors in a green space or having a window view are most effective, watching digital simulation of natural settings can provide significant benefits as well.

- **Nature improves vision.** Research suggests that in addition to providing a variety of visual stimuli, spending time viewing nature actually promotes healthy eye development and reduces myopic tendencies in children.

- **Nature promotes listening.** The harshness of loud, artificial noise not only puts children in a constant state of arousal, but it can also harm them. In contrast, natural sounds are restorative and promote auditory processing skills that can help children develop better communication skills in the context of social interactions.

- **Nature enhances touch.** Nature promotes exposure to varied tactile experiences that can help children enhance their sense of touch. Tolerance to a variety of tactile stimulation includes being able to walk barefoot, play in the dirt and mud, and even complete craft projects involving clay, glue, and paint.

- **Nature enhances taste and smell.** The crunch of a fresh picked apple. The scent of honeysuckle on the vine. Nature provides the richest of tastes and scents that enhance even the pickiest palate.

Seed Pods

Nature is made up of a variety of elements, such as water, soil, and sand. Each of these elements feels differently to the touch. For example, water can feel wet and "swooshy," soil can feel moist and soft, and sand can feel grainy and velvety. In this activity, you will work with a variety of elements to make seed pods, which are small balls that you can plant wherever you want the seeds to grow. By rolling the wet soil or clay, you allow your body to learn how to appreciate and experience the feeling of these different textures and surfaces.

Preparation
- Water
- Soil or clay
- Seeds of choice

Instructions
1. Combine a small amount of water, soil, or clay, and the seeds you want to plant. You may want to choose flower seeds that are bright and native to your area. Sunflowers or wildflowers are easy to grow and produce beautiful flowers. Or, you can choose vegetable seeds that will grow vegetables.

2. Once you have mixed together the soil/clay, water, and seeds, form the mixture into small balls and let them dry. It may take a few days for the seed pods to dry completely.

3. Then, take your seed pods home, and bury them wherever you want plants to grow!

Twirling

It is so important to move your body, and twirling around in circles is a fun way to do this! Not only is twirling fun, but it helps you with your balance and body awareness. When you twirl and twist, you activate the receptors in your inner ear that help you keep your balance. You are also teaching your body to discover where it stands in relation to others. This activity will help you pay attention to the movements of your body and develop your sense of balance as you practice twirling in circles.

Find an area, either indoors or outdoors, that provides you with enough space to move around. Stand with your arms stretched out, or at your sides, and spin around in a circle. After twirling around for a while, note how your body feels and answer the following questions.

How do you feel?

_____

_____

When you stop spinning, what does your body feel like?

_____

_____

Are you able to walk a straight line? Is there anything you have to do to keep your balance?

_____

_____

3D Artscape

In this activity, you'll be creating a three-dimensional work of art using a variety of items that you collect from an outdoor area in nature, such as leaves, sticks, twigs, and rocks. Each of these items is different in shape, color, size, and even weight, and your body engages with them differently. Creating a work of art from these objects will help your body learn to manipulate different types of objects while making a wonderful artform that is as unique as you.

Preparation

- Paper
- Craft items (e.g., glue, scissors, ribbon)
- Small items collected from your environment (e.g., leaves, sticks, rocks, etc.)

Instructions

1. Find a space where you can work outdoors and look around you. Take in the area with your eyes. Remember, just as you "take in the space," the space takes in you! What do you see? What colors are visible?

2. Gather at least five small items from your surroundings. These items can be anything you want, such as leaves, sticks, rocks, or shells.

3. Now, using your imagination, take your objects and put them together in a way that is attractive and interesting to you. You may want to stack some items or scatter them across the paper. It doesn't matter how you place your chosen objects. It is your special work of art, and the manner in which you place these objects is up to you.

4. After you've created your artscape, answer the questions on the reflection worksheet to reflect on your creation.

3D Artscape Reflection

Look closely at your three-dimensional artscape. How do you feel when you look at it?

_____

_____

_____

Now, close your eyes and touch your artwork. How would you describe it? Do the items feel similar or different? Is there a smell to the items? Or a sound?

_____

_____

_____

Every piece of art describes something about the artist. What do you think this artwork says about you?

_____

_____

_____

Sound Mapping

Listening skills not only help us focus our attention, but they also help us figure out where our bodies are in relation to the sounds we hear. For example, if you hear the siren of a firetruck blaring in the distance, my guess is that you stop and try to figure out where it is coming from and where it is headed. Just as important is figuring out where *you* are in relation to the firetruck. You want to make sure you're not in the way! In this activity, you will learn to focus on listening to the sounds around you.

Preparation
- Large piece of paper
- Tape
- Cardboard
- Pencil

Instructions
1. Find a safe place outdoors and position a large piece of paper in front of you. Tape the paper to a wall (if there is one nearby) or to a piece of cardboard so that it won't move.

2. With a pencil in hand, close your eyes, and begin to map the sounds you hear onto the paper in front of you. Perhaps you hear birds chirping in the right corner of the paper. Draw (symbolically) what that sounds like. Then, maybe you might hear the sound of rustling leaves in the trees overhead. Draw that sound on your paper too.

3. Map the sounds around you in symbolic shapes, lines, and zigzags to create a picture of this sound symphony.

4. When you're finished, open your eyes and give your map a title. Then, reflect on your experience of creating the sound map using the questions on the reflection worksheet.

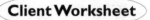

Sound Mapping Reflection

What was it like to listen to your surroundings?

It felt very peaceful are relaxing and allowed me to only focus on te sounds in my surroundings.

Were some sounds easier to recognize and draw out than others?

Birds tweeting is easy to recognize because of te sound they make, Drawing a bird is more complicated to draw compared to te leaf I drew,

How well did your drawing capture the sounds you heard?

I think my drawing capture te sounds I heard pretty well,

Sound Scape Story

In this activity, you will continue your work with the sound map. Our sensory system not only helps us navigate our world, but it also helps us discover how we fit in with and connect to the world around us. This exercise will invite you to create a story of how you fit in with the nature sounds that are around you.

Using the sound map that you created in the previous exercise, create a picture by connecting the various symbols you drew to depict the sounds. Then, tell a story about this picture, using the title you gave your sound map as a guide. What story is the artwork telling? Use the following space to write that story.

My artwork represents the transition of seasons. The leaf shows how it is falling from the tree which represents that it is changing to Fall. The bird in the tree helps to represent animals in Nature, as the bird watches the surroundings around him change. The story I am trying to tell helps show that things will change but you have to just keep going and adjust to the changes just like the bird, as well as, other animals have to.

Group Fun:
Sensory Swamp Quest

Going on a sensory swamp quest is a wonderful group activity that recruits a variety of senses, and it also promotes team building and problem solving. In this activity, children experience a variety of stimuli while blindfolded, and they must rely only on their other senses and their peers to guide them out of the "swamp."

Preparation

- Space to move (either indoors or outdoors)
- Blindfold
- Varied sensory bins, nature sounds, and aromatherapy scents
- A map of the space with a final destination
- A walking stick (optional)

Instructions

Instruct everyone to take off their shoes and socks. Choose one child in the group to be blindfolded, while the rest of the group serves as that child's "guide." The children who are guides help lead the barefoot and blindfolded child by providing descriptive directions through and around the "swamp." Sensory bins can be added for fun, inviting the blindfolded child to touch items in the bins as he or she is guided along the path.

For example, a bin filled with sand or seashells may be set along the path to suggest the direction is leading toward the beach and out of the swamp. Additionally, you can use nature recordings of seagulls, monkeys, or mooing cows to guide the blindfolded child out of the swamp and toward the "beach," "jungle," or "pasture," respectively.

The group can encourage the blindfolded child to follow these animal sounds toward the designated destination. Once the child reaches the final destination, have the group send another peer out to the "swamp."

After each child has had a turn being blindfolded, ask the group to reflect on the exercise using the questions on the reflection worksheet.

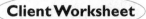

Sensory Swamp Quest Reflection

What was it like to be blindfolded? Barefoot?

_____

_____

What was it like to try to get through and out of the swamp?

_____

_____

Were the "guides" helpful in their descriptions? Was there anything that would have been more helpful?

_____

_____

What was it like when it was your turn to be a guide?

_____

_____

What did you learn about your senses? Which sense was the strongest? Which one needs more practice?

_____

_____

Nature-Informed Tactile Bins

It is important for children to experiment with a variety of sensory textures because it helps their body become more comfortable with different elements, and it helps them integrate their feelings regarding various tactile stimuli.

One way to help children experience a variety of textures in a fun and creative way is to create nature-informed tactile bins. To create these bins, find several containers of varying sizes, such as recycled plastic containers with lids, and place a variety of substances in the containers. Make sure to include items of differing textures, shapes, and sizes, such as feathers, sand, rocks, pebbles, sticks, shells, sea glass, dirt, tree bark, or water.

Invite children to close their eyes (or keep them open but don't peak in the container) and take turns touching the objects in the bins. It's important to allow children to engage with the bins in a fun, rather than a forced, manner. This can be done in a playful way by making a guessing game of the experience. Ask them to describe what they feel and to guess what each substance is. For example, are some items soft? Smooth? Prickly? Were there some items that felt nice or some that they didn't like to touch? Some children may find that touching some textures is uncomfortable and possibly repulsive. Always allow children to pass if they feel any discomfort.

After giving children some time to guess what is inside each container, allow them to remove some of the substances to reveal the contents. Children can return the substances to their respective containers once they have had time to interact with each substance. Giving children frequent opportunities to interact with the sensory bins will promote greater comfort and confidence in exploring varied tactile stimulation.

Analysis of Sensory Behaviors: Planning Worksheet

Student Name: _____

Therapist/Teacher: _____

School: _____   Date: _____

List behaviors:	List sensory system(s) involved:	Can the environment be changed? How?	Longer lasting sensory tasks:	Mini sensory tasks:	Sensory structured routines:

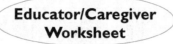

Sensory Diet Plan

Student Name: _____   School: _____

Date: _____   Therapist/Teacher: _____

Purpose: To help the child achieve a calm, organized state so he or she is ready to accept academic challenges in the classroom. A sensory diet is a scheduled routine that happens every day at about the same time.

Large sensory breaks help keep this student in an organized state for longer periods of time.

Mini sensory breaks help with fidgeting and changing the student's mood or state.

Mini breaks should be implemented in the class between the larger sensory breaks.

These sensory activities should not be used as rewards or consequences for behaviors. A separate behavior plan may need to be developed and implemented. Please consult with the occupational therapist for changes and modifications to this sensory diet.

Precautions:

Do not perform sensory activities if the child is sick.

Do not perform sensory activities if the child complains of pain or fatigue.

Closely supervise the child to prevent injuries.

Use your best judgment at all times!

Large sensory break ideas:

- _____

- _____

- _____

- _____

- _____

- _____

Mini sensory break ideas:

- _____
- _____
- _____
- _____
- _____
- _____

chapter
FIVE

Mindfulness and Nature-Based Tools for Creativity

"Conditions for creativity are to be puzzled; to concentrate; to accept conflict and tension; to be born everyday; to feel a sense of self."

— Erich Fromm

CREATIVITY AND DEVELOPMENT

Creativity has been defined as "the innate quest for originality" (Wilson, 2017, p. 3). It reflects the "ability to see patterns in the universe, to detect hidden links between what is and what could be" (Louv, 2012, p. 33). Creativity is also the cornerstone of innovation, as creative expression promotes the development of novel ideas and encourages openness to different perspectives. **Creativity is the ability to use our imagination to come up with something new and unique, whereas innovation involves putting this imagination into action.** Innovation channels creative flow by transcending the constraints of traditional ideas and converting creativity into something actionable.

Importantly, the development of creativity is founded in the context of early childhood learning and play (Banning & Sullivan, 2011). The ability to think of possibilities and in novel ways is the foundation of play and learning in childhood. Children learn by engaging with their environment, where there is a mutual interaction between the child and the setting. For example, the process of learning to walk not only consists of the development of gross motor skills and muscle movement, but it also involves creatively planning how to navigate the obstacles that may be in the way. My own daughters were "Houdinis" when it came to escaping their cribs when they were toddlers.

Additionally, creativity is associated with the development of unconventional thinking, which can help children transcend traditional rules and norms. For example, Carrie, a 10-year-old girl, was overheard during a slumber party inviting her friends to discuss their religious beliefs and political ideas. Concerned, her mother interrupted the discussion, admonishing Carrie for discussing politics and religion in the presence of "polite company." When Carrie asked why it was impolite to discuss these topics, her mother replied, "Because people get very upset when we talk about these issues." Carrie thought a moment and responded, "Well, maybe we should listen rather than talk."

Although fostering creativity is still considered a valuable component of childhood education, opportunities for creative thinking have diminished in early childhood learning programs as a result of an increased focus on purely academic skills and standardized testing instead (Baer, 2016; Baer & Kaufman, 2012; Beghetto, 2013; Russo, 2013). For example, in the current educational

67

system, children are tasked with finding one "correct" answer to a problem and are deterred from examining alternative solutions. Similarly, in learning environments that place greater value on academic performance, imaginative outdoor play has largely been replaced by indoor, adult-directed learning experiences (Gray, 2012).

These changes have had profound effects on the development of creative thinking in young children, as children are becoming less imaginative, less verbally expressive, and less able to see alternative views than previous generations (Gray, 2012). For example, creativity researcher Kyung Hee Kim examined data from over 200,000 children, ranging from kindergarten through high school, who had taken the Torrance Tests of Creative Thinking and found that creative thinking scores have steadily declined since 1990. This decrease was most significant for children in kindergarten through third grade. One possible reason for this decline is the increased emphasis on conformity in thinking in the school system (e.g., standardized tests) and a reduction in free time. According to Kim, "Hurried lifestyles and a focus on academics and enrichment activities have led to over-scheduling structured activities and academic-focused programs [...] at the expense of playtime" (2011, p. 293).

In this accelerated academic educational format, children are becoming increasingly unfamiliar with how to "pretend," and are needing instruction on how to play (Russo, 2013). Because contemporary early childhood learning experiences emphasize academic learning and school readiness, they diminish opportunities for play-based learning that promote critical thinking and creative expression. Children are struggling to enter into the realm of make-believe as they look for the logical "right" answers. You can test this out yourself. Place miniature animals and people, or puppets, in front of young children and ask them to tell you a story. Increasingly, children are deferring to the adult, "I don't know, what story do you want to tell?"

According to researcher and psychology professor at Boston University, Peter Gray (2012), "creativity is nurtured by freedom and stifled by the continuous monitoring, evaluation, adult-direction, and pressure to conform that restrict children's lives today." Therefore, in the current learning environment—where there is an excessive push for academic enrichment and children are deprived of outdoor time due to safety concerns about vigorous play—kids are spending more and more time in sedentary activities instead of engaging in creative play. We need to let kids be kids! Children need to have more free, unplugged, and unstructured time at home and school. They need opportunities for nondirective play in sensory-rich environments that invite and inspire innovation, expression, and creativity.

NATURE AND CREATIVITY: PROCESS OR PRODUCT?

Creativity is both a process and a product. It is an interaction whereby we are both shaping, and shaped by, the process (Atkins & Snyder, 2018). As young children, we are able to sing, draw, dance, and make art without fear of judgment. However, somewhere along the way, we are told that "cows are not purple" and "skies must be blue," and we doubt our ability to be creative. We internalize these criticisms, sabotaging our innate curiosities and creative expression. This results in the silencing of the budding singer, the grounding of the apprentice dancer, and immobilization of the novice painter who stares at a blank canvas. Children's ability to attempt new and different activities becomes squelched as they anticipate their failure at "doing it right." Our miniature "Einsteins" become shackled by rules and criticisms.

Creativity can only be fostered when we do not squelch it with judgment or restrictive experiences (Atkins & Snyder, 2018). It is for this reason that nature is the ultimate teacher for creative expression, as it inspires and encourages expression without criticism. It recognizes the power of the process over the product. For example, young children who are not restricted in their efforts will spend hours interacting in the natural surroundings through imaginary play and scientific experimentation. Rain puddles become fodder for experimentation as children test their reasoning around questions such as, "What happens when I jump into the puddle?" Soil and water combine to make a clay worthy of primitive pottery. Stacked snowballs form a fortress against the wintery winds. Without the freedom to examine and explore all possibilities, discovery and innovation would yield to existing theory, and the world would remain flat! **Children are little naturalists, and when we do not provide them with opportunities to creatively interact with nature, we are hindering future generations of scientists, physicians, architects, mathematicians, musicians, and poets.**

NATURE AND METAPHOR: WHEN WORDS AREN'T ENOUGH

Not only does nature provide a forum through which children can create and innovate, it also is a way in which they can construct (and reconstruct) life experiences. Childhood is filled with experiences that lack or transcend language, and nature provides a medium from which children can make meaning out of these circumstances. For example, comprehension of death or life, as well as awe and wonder, are difficult to capture with words. Nature can be that medium that promotes creative expression without words. When engaging in natural settings, there is an interconnection that occurs between the medium (nature) and the artist (child). The child does not force the expression but engages in a collaborative relationship with the environment, in turn bringing forth what the natural elements are wanting to convey and perhaps giving rise to a shared story.

For example, I was working with a 16-year-old teenage boy who presented with anxiety. He was telling me about his latest camping trip and began to describe the river that he had encountered. He described how "she moved swiftly, rushing strewn leaves and branches around bends, until they abruptly halted at a gathering of twigs. Then, the river bid adieu to the debris and resumed her journey down the winding path." The story created by this young man around his encounter with a river became a metaphor for his journey with anxiety as he moved smoothly along his life and then experienced a stumbling block that seemed to sabotage his forward movement. However, it was only a temporary stop, leaving behind that which no longer served him and allowing him to resume his life. While his experience with anxiety escaped his vocabulary, the metaphor of the river captured it poetically. It enhanced his ability to understand his relationship with anxiety and the river itself.

When children intentionally engage with nature, it also provides them a creative platform through which they can restructure their life stories (Campbell, 1991). It allows them to recreate the narrative surrounding their perceived reality and create a "new and preferable reality" that is empowering and promotes meaning-making (Lahad, 2006). For example, a child who has been told that she is "no good" and "lazy" can restructure this inherited tale by (perhaps) tending to a community garden. By digging in the dirt, pulling weeds (a metaphor for getting rid of that which stifles growth), and watering the garden, this child recreates her story from one in which she is viewed as "lazy" to one in which she is capable of doing physically demanding work. She also benefits from seeing how her hard work results in the growth of tiny sprouts followed by beautiful plants.

Another wonderful example of how nature allows children to construct (and reconstruct) their life circumstances is Tikkun Farm, which is an urban farm in Cincinnati that serves the local community of underserved minority children and refugees. The farm's mission is to heal individuals by repairing communities and restoring nature. In addition to many other great programs, each summer they hold a farm camp that allows for children of all ages to have a farm immersion experience. Children tend to the animals, including the alpacas, and learn to make fiber arts from the fleece of the animals. They prepare (and eat) a farm-to-table meal. They learn to be in communion with animals, nature, and other individuals who do not look, speak, or live like them. Some children may help around the farm by gathering eggs, watering young apple trees, and tending to a sick chicken, while others assist in harvesting from the garden and preparing a community dinner. In addition, children are encouraged to be expressive through art, music, dance, and writing, and they learn about different cultures through creative arts and food.

Tikkun Farm is a powerful and profound program where stories of re-storying personal narratives are common. The children interact with creative intention in nature and learn how to live in a diverse community with respect, generosity, trust, and radical hospitality. It is a prime example of how nature promotes creative expression and allows children to make meaning by (re)constructing their life narratives. Children who are otherwise subject to the social prescriptions of living in an inner city (e.g., poverty, lack of privilege, crime) are able to experience the equality offered by working with other children from diverse backgrounds as they tend to the farm, feed the animals, harvest vegetables, and make and share meals together. Working collaboratively to complete these tasks challenges stereotypes and promotes exposure to diverse thinking and the liberation of diverse expression. The children are no longer alien to one another but, rather, a community of creative diversity. This experience of intentional creative collaboration inspires children to view themselves and their communities beyond the neighborhood block in which they live.

The following case study, which is adapted from the work of Ronen Berger and John McLeod (2006), further exemplifies how nature provides a creative outlet through which children can make meaning out of their life circumstances. It also illustrates how nature serves as a collaborative partner in the therapeutic process.

Case Study

JOSEPH

Joseph, a 12-year-old boy, experienced communication problems and social difficulties. He was not comfortable in the counseling room, so his therapist invited him to go for walks just outside his classroom. Over time, the parameter of the walks expanded to a nearby riverbank, where Joseph always gravitated toward the same spot, under a willow tree. Given that the goal of therapy was to increase Joseph's social and communication skills, these nature sessions began with Joseph and his therapist engaging in a familiar activity together, such as brewing tea over a fire. Through the repetitions of these activities, the relationship between Joseph and his therapist slowly grew as they navigated the natural surroundings in this "sacred space."

As the sessions continued, Joseph continued to return with his therapist to this same location, where it became evident that he was constructing a small barrier around the "tea ceremony" area using sticks and stones that he had collected. When the barrier was complete, Joseph's use of language expanded to include him wanting to talk about his internal world. He began sharing more about his thoughts and feelings, and felt more comfortable disclosing memories and tales from his daily life encounters. When winter approached and the weather prevented sessions from occurring outdoors, therapy resumed indoors. However, it was noted that when Joseph would experience any difficulties, he would lead his therapist back to the place on the riverbank, which he had named "Home in Nature." According to Berger and McLeod (2006):

> "It was as though Joseph needed to check that the safe, sacred space that he and his therapist had physically built together, a space that also symbolized their therapeutic alliance, was still there. It seemed like he wanted to see what had changed during the season and what needed to be reconstructed." (p. 83)

Providing Joseph with the opportunity to use his inherent connection to nature and his innate creative expression enabled him to become more expansive in his language expression and promoted the cultivation of a deep, trusting relationship with his therapist. Prior to beginning treatment, Joseph had been socially and verbally awkward. As Joseph was given the space to follow his natural expressiveness in creating a "Home in Nature," he began to feel safe. He was able to unleash his ability to effectively communicate with others and experience relationships in a meaningful way.

SUMMARY AND EXERCISES

Creativity is the catalyst for innovation and ingenuity, and children develop creativity through expressive play in sensory-rich environments. Children have an instinctual and innate response to the natural world and its beauty (Atkins & Snyder, 2018), and when children interact with nature, it invites exploration through the complexity of possibility. In addition, nature serves as a medium from which children can (re)construct and make meaning around life circumstances. For example, a butterfly can serve as a symbol of transcending hardships, an ant may signify the ability to work in a community and accomplish great feats, and the fidelity of the seasons reminds us that this moment is but a moment that will eventually pass. Nature illuminates the complexities of life while offering metaphors that promote creative expression and enhance meaning.

The following pages contain a variety of tools to help children reconnect with nature and cultivate their creative potential. The first handout, **Creativity and Nature**, provides caregivers and educators with a summary that explains how engaging in nature promotes creative expression, including how the use of metaphor can help children (re)construct their story and their reality. The worksheets and handouts that follow contain a variety of activities to promote children's creative interaction with nature. **Many of these activities are intended to allow children to express thoughts, ideas, and stories that they may be unable to put down in words.**

Creativity and Nature

Creative expression is essential for healthy development. It encourages children to be open to different perspectives, promotes the development of new ideas, and is the foundation for innovation. Importantly, creativity develops during early childhood through the context of unstructured, free play. Outdoor play in particular provides a multisensory environment that facilitates creative expression and innovation, as it is filled with a variety of challenges and conflict that children must overcome.

When we give children opportunities for nondirected, outdoor play, they can generate new ideas and ways of experiencing the world. Rain and dirt become ingredients for making mud pies, and wooden logs become unicorns that children can ride.

Unstructured, outdoor play not only promotes problem-solving skills and innovation, but it also gives children the ability to glean novel perspectives around such things as the temporariness of rain or sunshine and the discomfort of a cold day.

Not only is nature the best teacher for creative innovation, but it also allows for meaning-making as children construct (and reconstruct) their life circumstances. Nature represents a safe outlet through which children can creatively express what they can't put into words.

For example, the transformation of a caterpillar to a butterfly sets the stage for a discussion around beliefs pertaining to death, dying, and the afterlife. The molting of a snake's skin may spark discussion around the transformative changes that occur during puberty. Watching the collaborative work of ants building a hill can represent the power of teamwork. Tree seedlings sprouting around an old tree trunk demonstrate the continuation of life and legacy.

Seasons in nature become metaphors for seasons in life. Nature is filled with tales of courage, collaboration, and compassion that help inform the human story.

Nature Print

Being able to express yourself creatively is so important for healthy growth and development. It helps you identify new ideas and solutions to problems, and it allows you to express your thoughts and feelings in different ways. In this activity, you'll use your creativity to collaborate with nature in making a nature print T-shirt, which contains a bunch of different shapes and patterns created from different items found in nature.

Preparation

- T-shirt
- Fabric paint
- Paintbrushes
- Nature items (e.g., leaves, flower petals)

Instructions

1. Go on a nature walk and find four to five items that you want to use to print on your shirt. Choose a variety of items that differ in shape, size, and texture. For example, you might choose an item as small as a shamrock or as big as a palm frond. The choice is yours!

2. Using your paintbrush, paint each nature item so that it is completely covered with paint on one side. While the paint is wet, press the nature item onto your T-shirt so that it leaves an imprint on the shirt.

3. Carefully lift the nature item off the shirt, and discard it if you are finished using it for this project.

4. Repeat this process with all the other nature items you collected, painting and pressing, until you are satisfied with your T-shirt.

5. Put on your nature T-shirt and reflect on your creation using the questions on the reflection worksheet.

Nature Print Reflection

What was it like to go and pick out your nature objects?

_____

_____

_____

Did you choose any specific leaves or flowers? Do these have special meaning?

_____

_____

_____

What kinds of patterns did you make on your shirt?

_____

_____

_____

Reflect on your project and the process of making your shirt. How were you feeling at that time?

_____

_____

_____

Do you feel differently now? How so?

_____

_____

_____

Nature provides us with a beautiful way to express ourselves. What does your project say about you?

_____

_____

_____

Nature Sculpture

Sculptures are four-dimensional artifacts that tell a story. In this activity, you will create a sculpture using items that you have found from nature. This activity will allow you to think creatively about the items you select and how they fit together in new ways. First, find a variety of nature items that you can use to create your sculpture, such as rocks, feathers, sticks, seashells, dried seaweed, or dried flowers.

As you collect these items, take the time to look at each item and notice its unique qualities. For example, is it hard or soft? Wet or dry? Stiff or flexible? Then, create a sculpture by gluing these items together. As you create your sculpture, notice what it is like to bring these different items together and see how they interact. When you are done, give your sculpture a name and answer the following questions.

What objects did you select? Why?

_____

_____

_____

What was it like putting the objects together? Were some things harder than others to connect? Why?

_____

_____

_____

What did you name the sculpture? Why?

_____

_____

_____

What story does it tell?

_____

_____

_____

Nature Staining

Have you ever written with a bark pencil? Did you know that freshly fallen stems will write with green stain? In this activity, you'll create a work of art using nature as your paint. Go for a walk and pick up any nature items you can find that have a stain. These can be juicy berries, green sticks, or dark pieces of nuts and bark—anything with pigment that you can use to write or draw.

Choose your items and draw or write in the following space. There are no rules, just let your imagination lead you.

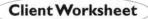

Mud Art

The creation of mud is as unique as the soil and water that is mixed together. Sandy soil will produce a grainier mud, while sooty soil will produce mud that is very dark and smooth.

In this activity, you'll creatively express yourself by making mud art. Find some dirt that you'd like to use, and mix it with some water until it becomes the consistency of paint. You may want to experiment with different types of dirt to make all kinds of mud "paint." When you're done mixing the mud together, dip a paintbrush into the "paint" and spread it across the paper. You may want to use different size paintbrushes or even try painting with sticks. Or, maybe you want to finger paint and feel the mud between your fingers. It doesn't matter. This is a creation among you, the mud, and the paper. When you're done creating your mud art, answer the following questions.

What soil(s) did you choose? What kind of mud did it make?

_____

_____

What did you use to paint? How did you choose?

_____

_____

What did it feel like to paint with the mud?

_____

_____

What would you name your painting? Why? What story does it tell?

_____

_____

Shadow Drawing

A shadow is an impression of a shape against light. In this activity, you'll be creating a picture using shadows of objects that you find outside. To complete your shadow drawing, you'll need to intentionally collaborate with the sun to create different shadows. As you work with the sun, think about what creative ways you can cast shadows onto your paper and how you can create different patterns and shapes.

Preparation

- Sunny space
- Paper
- Tape
- Nature objects (e.g., leaves, feathers, shells)
- Colored pencils, paint, chalk, or crayons

Instructions

1. Find a sunny space where you can tape a piece of paper to a wall (or vertical flat surface) to keep it secure.

2. Identify objects from nature that you want to use in your art creation. These can be seashells, rocks, feathers, leaves, or anything else that you might like to use.

3. Place your nature object(s) between the sun and the paper so that it creates a shadow on the paper. Outline the shadow of the object.

4. Once you've finished drawing shadow outlines, feel free to decorate your shadow drawing by adding color or texture to it. For example, maybe you want to glue sand onto the paper to give it some texture or draw with crayons to add a pop of color. Complete the drawing in any way that you'd like.

5. Once you've completed your shadow drawing, answer the questions on the reflection worksheet.

Shadow Drawing Reflection

What objects did you choose? Why?

_____

_____

_____

What was it like to work with the sun to create your drawing?

_____

_____

_____

What did you add to the drawing to enhance it (e.g., color, texture)? Why?

_____

_____

_____

What did you name your drawing? What story does it tell?

_____

_____

_____

Mandala (Circle Art)

A mandala is a geometric design that is usually in the shape of a circle. In some cultures, the mandala is a very special circle that is considered sacred. In this activity, you will practice creating a mandala using nature and a circle of your choice. How you create your mandala art is up to you as the artist. Let your mandala tell a story that is special to you.

Find some objects outside that you can use to create your mandala, such as sand, feathers, sticks, small shells, nuts, flower petals, or leaves. Then, create an outline of a circle that is large enough to fill with your selected objects. You can draw a circle in chalk on the concrete, or on a piece of cardboard or sturdy paper. You can also use colored sand to outline your circle. You may even want to draw a circle inside a shoebox so that your objects can stay secure in the box after you are finished. It doesn't matter as long as it is a place where you can draw a circle. Arrange the objects you are using in a way that feels good to you. Let the objects guide you in creating the story in the circle. When you are finished, give your mandala a name and answer the following questions.

What objects did you choose? Why?

_____

_____

How did you feel making your mandala?

_____

_____

What story did you create with your mandala?

_____

_____

What did you name it?

_____

_____

Sand Art

Sand comes in many different textures and colors. For example, some types of sand feel rough and grainy, while others feel smooth and powdery. Sand also differs in color, depending on where it is found. On different beaches all across the world, sand can be orange, black, red, gold, white, green, or even pink! In this activity, you'll layer different color sand on top of each other to create a beautiful expressive piece of art. As you create layers with all these different colors, it will begin to make a unique design that is special to you.

Preparation

- Different colors of sand
- Clear container (e.g., Tupperware bin, plastic bottle)
- Toothpick or wooden skewer
- Funnel (optional)

Instructions

1. Find a clear container you can use to create your sand art. If you're using a container that has a narrow opening, like a bottle, it is helpful to use a funnel to pour the sand into the container.

2. Take a moment to look at your sand and think about what colors you want to use. Is there a certain color that you like best today? Pick a color that you'd like to start with.

3. Look at your container and imagine the sand flowing into the container. Is a pattern emerging in your thoughts?

4. Slowly let a little bit of sand flow into the container, and then stop. Before adding any more sand, think about whether you want to use another color or continue with the same color.

5. You can even use a toothpick (or wooden skewer for containers with longer openings) to push down on the sand and create a dip.

6. Keep alternating colors and "dips" until your container is filled.

7. Look at the design you have created. What does it look like to you? Give your project a name.

Group Fun:
Guerilla Rock Art

In recent years, rock art has become an eco-creative way to spread messages around the world. People are painting meaningful and creative messages on rocks and sharing them in communities, parks, and gardens—anywhere that an eco-message is welcomed.

This activity encourages children to cultivate meaningful ideas and share them in an innovative manner with others. Additionally, children may experience a creative way to connect with others through the exchange of rock messages.

Help children create their own guerilla rock art by gathering a variety of rocks that they can decorate for this activity. Smooth and flat rocks work best.

Invite children to decorate their rocks any way that they want. While children are creating their rock art, ask them what messages they'd like to convey on their rocks, where they want to share these messages, and why these messages are important to them.

Then, as a group, go for a walk and find places to leave these rocks that need beauty.

I have found rocks that look like ladybugs in Central Park, happy faces on rocks near my neighborhood swimming pool, and painted rocks with inspirational messages sitting on park benches, in gardens, or at the beach. Invite children to use their imagination!

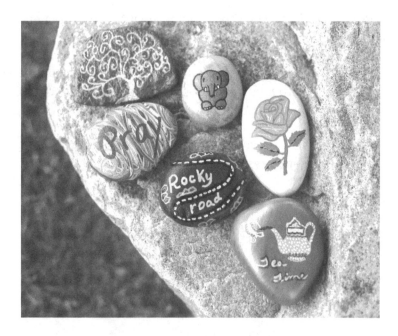

chapter
SIX

Nature-Based Mindfulness, Trauma, and Resiliency

"A bird sitting on a tree is never afraid of the branch breaking, because her trust is not on the branch but on its wings."

— Unknown

In our current society, children are experiencing trauma at profound rates, with research suggesting that almost half of children—approximately 35 million—have experienced some sort of traumatic event by the age of 16 (NSCH, 2011/2012). These adverse childhood experiences are wide-ranging and can include physical, sexual, and emotional abuse; neglect; domestic violence; natural disasters; terrorism; and community violence. Not surprisingly, these traumatic experiences can have enduring negative effects on children's physical and emotional development. In particular, the findings of the groundbreaking Adverse Childhood Experiences (ACE) study found that exposure to traumatic events in childhood increases the risk for physical disease and disorder, including cancer, heart disease, and diabetes, and is also associated with lifelong psychological distress (Felitti et al., 1998). Children who are exposed to multiple adverse experiences are at particular risk for negative physical and mental health outcomes (Hughes et al., 2017).

Therefore, when working with children and issues of trauma, it is imperative to have a foundational understanding of how trauma impacts development and to utilize trauma-informed practices that help children navigate these traumatic experiences. In this chapter, I'll explore these negative effects of trauma in greater detail and discuss how engaging with nature represents one avenue of treatment that can promote children's resilience and recovery.

IMPACT OF TRAUMA ON DEVELOPMENT

When children are exposed to threat and their body perceives danger, the body undergoes a series of physiological changes that prepare the body to respond. In particular, the sympathetic nervous system becomes activated, releasing a flood of stress hormones into the body (e.g., cortisol, adrenaline, norepinephrine) and signaling the limbic system to "turn on." These changes represent what is referred to as the fight, flight, or freeze response because they mobilize the body to respond to the threat at hand.

While these changes are adaptive in the context of real danger, children who have been traumatized by adverse childhood experiences can get "stuck" in this chronic state of hyperarousal. It's as if their fight, flight, or freeze response is in a state of constant activation. As a result, children can be easily triggered by situations that bring up memories of the trauma. For example, I once worked with a 7-year-old girl living with a foster family, who became completely paralyzed with fear whenever she heard adults disagreeing. The interactions did not need to be aggressive or abusive for her to shrivel into a corner in the fetal position. She could not articulate why she was so afraid; she just instinctively responded to the situation. It was later discovered that her birth parents had a tumultuous relationship that often resulted in loud screaming matches and things being thrown against the wall (and at each other), and the girl was put in the middle of these arguments as leverage. She had been emotionally and physically unsafe when adults disagreed, and, in turn, her brain registered every argument as dangerous, and her body responded by shutting down.

In addition to chronic hypervigilance, trauma can also affect children by resulting in symptoms of dissociation. Specifically, children may "zone out" or dissociate to mentally detach from any situations, images, or thoughts that remind them of the trauma. As a result, they may appear inattentive in class or at home. They may also develop new fears or experience intense anxiety, causing them to be more prone to self-harm behavior and emotional outbursts. Similarly, they may be plagued with nightmares as their brains attempt to process the traumatic events. When such interruptions in sleep occur, children may experience difficulties concentrating, appear lethargic, or fall asleep in the middle of the day.

Additionally, because many children do not have the language to articulate their feelings or fears, they may report a variety of somatic complaints, such as headaches, stomachaches, or nonspecific pain in parts of the body. On the other hand, for children who are more verbal, exposure to trauma may cause an increase in thoughts or discussions related to death and dying. Children who are exposed to traumatic deaths, in particular, may pose questions around this topic. For example, while running a group for marginalized middle-school children, I became acutely aware of the threats faced by these children on a daily basis. They would return to the group following a weekend filled with gun violence, drug busts, and suicides. I was appalled at how matter-of-fact the discussions were around these traumatic events and the subsequent thoughts around death and dying.

RESILIENCY AND TRAUMA RECOVERY

The effects of trauma on childhood development are so profound because trauma negatively impacts the way in which children's brains are hardwired. Children who have experienced trauma experience changes in the neural pathways that influence how they perceive and respond to the world. In particular, trauma leads them to perceive the world as threatening and to respond to it as such. However, children are resilient, and even after a traumatic event, they can recover. Their bodies and brains are built for restoration and resiliency. Childhood is a period characterized by rapid development and growth, and the brain in particular has the most plasticity during this period, meaning that it is malleable and can form new neural pathways. The brain's ability to rewire itself is known as "neuroplasticity," and it explains why treatment can correct any faulty pathways that have been formed as a result of trauma.

Utilizing the brain's natural capacity for neuroplasticity, treatment for trauma consists of a combination of approaches. The first approach (top down) involves talking, reconnecting with others, and processing the traumatic event. The second approach (bottom up) involves engaging the body fully by providing it with experiences of empowerment, strength, and confidence that differ from that of the trauma (van der Kolk, 2015). Too often, however, we rely solely on top-down approaches by utilizing talk therapy and cognitive processing as our only interventions for trauma. This dismisses the library of memories catalogued among the sensory organs, hypothalamic-pituitary-adrenal axis, and musculoskeletal systems. In addition, trauma in early childhood often never reaches the part of the brain used in speech (RB-Banks & Meyer, 2017). All the systems of the body are impacted by trauma, and memories are stored in the body (not just the brain), making it difficult for children to recount traumatic memories.

Therefore, clinicians cannot rely on talk therapy as the sole form of treatment. Rather, early childhood trauma must be processed through more physical means, including those available in the various expressive therapies, such as art, drama, play, dance, and movement therapy (RB-Banks & Meyers, 2017). Ultimately, children need to experience their bodies and sensory organs in a safe way. "For real change to take place, the body needs to learn that the danger has passed and to live in the reality of the present" (van der Kolk, 2015, p. 21). **To capitalize on the body's capacity for resiliency, we need to engage children in whole-brain, whole-body experiences that directly address the trauma and promote agency, and nature therapy is one such approach that provides these experiences.**

NATURE THERAPY AND BUILDING RESILIENCY

Nature therapy promotes resiliency and, in turn, recovery from trauma in a number of ways. Most notably, engaging in nature acts as a buffer to traumatic events because it provides children with experiences that foster the development of a unique set of coping skills. According to the *Basic Ph* (*b*elief, *a*ffect, *s*ocial *i*magination, *c*ognition, and *ph*ysiological) model, the unique combination of six different coping styles helps children persevere in the face of adversity and reduces the negative impact of trauma on development (Lahad, Shacham, & Ayalon, 2013). Engaging in nature nurtures these key elements of resiliency.

First, engaging with nature helps children make meaning out of the trauma by allowing them to construct and reconstruct the trauma narrative (*belief*). Nature-informed interventions allow children to reconnect with themselves and others in a complex and unpredictable manner that encourages creative and playful engagement, which results in agency and meaning-making. Children are empowered to craft meaningful narratives about themselves and the trauma. When they strategize how to climb a tree or maneuver a log bridge over a creek, they can create and act out stories that allow them to confront their fears and build confidence. While they were unable to stop the traumatic event, children can develop mastery around other difficulties found in nature, which strengthens their ability to problem solve in the face of life's challenges (*cognition*) and builds confidence in their physical body as they overcome these challenges (*physiological*).

In addition, the ionic exchange that occurs when interacting with the natural elements helps promote a calm and alert state (*affect*). When children intentionally interact with the natural elements, this encourages them to be fully present in the here-and-now, as opposed to reliving the past experience of the trauma or worrying about how it will impact them in the future. This reorienting effect of nature can help children bypass the defense mechanisms they use to distance themselves from the trauma (e.g., regression, acting out, dissociation) and ground them back to the present moment (Berger, 2016). For example, I will often utilize natural elements in my grounding exercises with children who experience dissociation or intrusive thoughts related to the trauma. I may have them hold a rock, a piece of sea glass, or a seashell and then have them describe the object they are holding in great detail. In addition to bringing their attention back to the present, the object may represent a happier or more peaceful time, which serves to interrupt any intrusive thought processes. The use of aromatherapy, sensory bins, or nature soundtracks are other ways to facilitate mindful interaction with nature and promote a calm state.

Moreover, nature inherently stimulates creativity and playfulness in children (*imagination*). When children are able to reconnect with their inner child and creative self, this aids in recovery and fosters growth as children engage in creative expression surrounding the trauma. For example, Berger and Lahad (2013) created a nature-informed program for the surviving children of war-torn Liberia, in which children narrated a story whereby they became the protectors of the forests that had been ravaged by the fires and destruction of war. They went into the woods, painted their faces with warrior paint, and took part in an induction ceremony that named them as Forest Guardians. The children then began to clean up the forest and create natural habitats and shelters for the animals that had been forced to leave the uninhabitable grounds. The children became empowered as they rewrote and reenacted a narrative of hope.

Finally, engaging with nature also provides children with a sense of support as they connect to the earth and its creatures (*social*). Plants and animals are responsive to our actions and interactions (Kahn & Kellert, 2002). The dynamic interactions that occur between children and nature are visible all around, such as when a young child intentionally waters a seedling and provides it with encouraging words to aid in its growth, or when a dog frantically wags its tail upon seeing a child approach. The social connection that nature provides is also exemplified through the emotional support animal, whose sole purpose is to provide companionship and aide to children during vulnerable situations, such as in courtrooms, medical offices, and airports. Interacting with the trees, plants, and animals opens up an expansive array of relationships that coexist within the day-to-day narrative of children, which widens their support network.

One of the most powerful examples of healing that I have experienced as a clinician is the story of Anna, a young girl who was sexually assaulted while walking home from school. Through her interaction with nature, Anna was able to rewrite her narrative, recover from the trauma, and reclaim her life. The following is her story.

Case Study
ANNA

Anna, a small-framed, 15-year-old Caucasian female, sat engulfed by the overstuffed chair in my office. She looked down, past the floor, to the day her world collapsed. She was walking home from school when three men jumped her, threw her against the huge old oak tree that lay on the outskirts of her family's farm and proceeded to rape her. They left her against the tree, with torn clothes, battered and forever changed.

After a time (how long, Anna could not recall), she walked home to her beloved lakeside farm that was just a quarter-mile from the assault. She described her home as her "safe place" where she was able to "just be myself," surrounded by her animals, which included horses, dogs, goats and chickens. After finishing her numerous chores around the farm, she would grab a book and take her kayak to the center of the lake, spending hours immersed in the narratives. This had been her haven...until now.

Anna's mother met her at the door, and Anna collapsed in her arms. The police were called but were unable to make sense of the traumatized youth's story and unintentionally violated her with their dismissal.

She was left feeling ashamed, alone and unlovable. She began isolating herself from her siblings, her friends and even her animals.

Anna's ability to discuss any aspect of her trauma was enhanced when Max, my therapy dog, joined the sessions. Initially, we would take Max for short walks around the practice neighborhood. On one of those walks, Anna proclaimed her love of kayaking and asked if we might be able to go one day. I had never taken a client kayaking before, and I was unsure of the liability and ethical ramifications. Still, Anna felt strongly that she wanted to go kayaking with me on our nearby creek.

Following consultation with several colleagues, I asked Anna's mother about the possibility of holding a session on the kayaks. To my surprise, Anna's mother enthusiastically agreed: "Anna is a very proficient kayaker and a very strong swimmer. I am happy to consent."

The following week, we met at the area where I keep my kayaks. Anna had brought her own. We put the kayaks in on the sandy shore of the lazy creek and paddled around for a while. Anna had become more animated since we took our sessions outdoors, and she eagerly pressed for us to move out of the calm water to the more challenging adjoining river. I decided that this was indicative of her trust in our relationship—to venture into deeper, more challenging waters.

As we entered the mouth of the river, I remembered the bulkhead that was just around the bend. I had frequently found myself paddling too close and instantly getting sucked into the undertow, which resulted in my kayak being thrust into a head-on collision with a rock barrier. I knew how to release from the undertow, but I was curious how my eager client would view the challenge.

As we paddled into the river, the waters began to churn, splashing in the wake of passing boats. Anna stayed safely in the middle of the river, while I deliberately ventured slightly closer to shore. Sure enough, the current grabbed my kayak and forced me against the rock bed. Anna remained safely beyond the current and was surprised to see me paddling against the waves and rocks. She called out to me, "Stop paddling! Just let the waves take you in…then release."

I acted as if I had not heard her wisdom and continued to struggle with the current. Finally, Anna yelled, "Stop fighting it, Dr. Cheryl! You have to let it take you in…to release you! You will be fine. Just let go!"

AH! YES! Don't fight it. Just release it! So, I did…and easily paddled to my very wise (and now frowning) client.

"You knew how to do that all along, didn't you? You were trying to show me that I need to not fight this thing so much, right?" She lowered her head and began to cry for the first time. We adjoined our paddles and for the rest of the session sat in silence in the middle of the river.

The weeks that followed were an emotional roller coaster filled with disclosure, tears and healing. At the end of one session, Anna announced, "It is time. It is time to return to the oak tree." She was ready to return to the place where her violation had occurred. To confront the oak tree that had stood witness. The sessions that followed were characterized by imagery and preparation for Anna's journey to the location of the assault.

Finally, she was ready. We met at the site of the rape. We got out of the car and slowly walked to the tree—a huge ancient oak whose branches, now bare preparing for the winter rest, stretched out, welcoming Anna. I could never have been prepared for what happened next. Anna ran to the tree, wrapped her arms around its wide girth and began to cry, "Thank you!"

Anna had now slipped to the base of the tree and continued, "Thank you! During everything, you stood with me. You held me up. You never left me!"

Anna's mother and I just looked at each other in astonishment. Anna was grateful to the oak tree for holding witness to her assault and remaining with her throughout the entire atrocity. Anna's rape is *remembered through, with and in the context of the land and seas, and air, and creatures.* She wanted to honor the old oak, so she planted bulbs at its base. In the early spring, Anna returned to find the most beautiful small white flowers peeking up through the late frost...a sign that life can hold beauty even after devastation. (Reprinted with permission, Fisher, 2017).

Anna reclaimed her life through the organic relationship developed with my co-therapist (Max), the mysteries found in the musings of a winding river, and the fidelity of an oak tree. Through her interaction with nature, Anna was able to rewrite her narrative and reclaim her life.

SUMMARY AND EXERCISES

Although the effects of trauma encompass the body, as well as the brain, engaging in the natural settings allows children to develop the necessary coping skills to buffer against the effects of trauma, develop self-confidence, and regain a sense of hope. **The pages that follow include a variety of mindfulness nature-based activities that promote confidence and mastery, along with empowerment and agency, so that children can draw on their capacity for resiliency and recover from trauma.** The first handout, **Nature-Based Mindfulness, Trauma, and Resiliency**, provides caregivers and educators with a brief summary that explains how trauma affects the brain, what behaviors may result, and how engaging in nature promotes coping skills that aid in recovery. The worksheets and handouts that follow contain activities that are intended to promote the development of coping skills for children who have experienced trauma, including grounding, self-soothing, creative expression, and empowerment exercises.

Nature-Based Mindfulness, Trauma, and Resiliency

Trauma and the Brain

Childhood trauma results in the activation of parts of the brain that signal danger to the entire body. Basically, the child's body perceives danger and prepares for an immediate fight, flight, or freeze response. Although this evolutionary response is adaptive in the face of danger, children who experience trauma can become "stuck" in this survival mode even after the danger has subsided. Therefore, it is not uncommon for children who have experienced trauma to exhibit the following behaviors:

- Hypervigilance
- Nightmares
- Decrease in concentration
- Increase in anxiety
- Insomnia

- Acting-out behaviors (e.g., anger or agitation)
- Dissociation or daydreaming
- Body aches and pains
- Increase in fearfulness

Nature and Resiliency

The human body and brain are designed to be resilient, and it is possible for children to recover in the aftermath of a trauma. Because trauma often bypasses the language part of the brain and is stored in the body, the process of recovery must involve the whole body—not just the brain. Therefore, successful treatment must include physical approaches (e.g., movement-based therapies), as well as cognitive approaches (e.g., talking through and processing the trauma).

Nature-informed interventions represent one particular approach that provides children with a whole-brain, whole-body experience needed to recover from trauma, as engaging with nature promotes the development of a unique set of coping skills that facilitate children's capacity for resiliency and recovery. In particular, interacting with the natural elements helps children make sense of the trauma, promotes a calm and alert state, provides them with a connection to the earth and its creatures, provides endless opportunities for creativity and imagination, promotes the development of problem-solving skills, and facilitates a sense of mastery as children work to navigate the earth's various terrains.

Nature-Enhanced Grounding Kit

One of the challenges of trauma recovery is the tendency to dissociate ("zone out") or experience flashbacks regarding the trauma, as opposed to staying in the here-and-now. Whenever you start to feel yourself disconnecting from the present moment, it can be helpful to have some tools to reorient you and *ground* you back to the present. You can include these tools as part of a grounding kit and use them the next time you are feeling "out of it" or need to bring yourself back to the present moment. You might want to consider even getting a container, like a small backpack, to carry around these items so you can easily access your grounding kit whenever you need to.

- **Essential oils:** Dab a bit on your hands, bring your hands to your nose, and inhale. Peppermint, lavender, jasmine, and a blend named Dharma are particularly effective.

- **Hard candy:** Slowly suck on the candy and enjoy its flavors. Cinnamon, root beer, and key lime are some nice varieties you can try.

- **Transitional object** (from Chapter 2): Hold your object and feel its shape. Notice its color and weight. Is it heavy or light? Smooth or rough? Gently rub it on your arm or leg.

- **Duck call or small whistle:** Take a deep breath and blow. Listen to the sound.

- **Nature cards** (see the Nature Cards activity sheet): Look through your nature cards and describe out loud what you see in the picture. Pay attention to the colors, shapes, and objects on the card.

Nature Cards

The brain helps us detach from bad memories and thoughts by zoning out. Although a little bit of zoning out and daydreaming is normal, too much can keep us from being fully present in the moment. One way to help bring yourself back to the present moment is to use grounding cards, which are an easy-to-access tool that you can use whenever you find that you are starting to disconnect from reality.

For this activity, you'll be creating grounding cards that are focused on images in nature that you find pleasing or relaxing.

To create your nature cards, find a camera you can use, or use the camera feature on your cell phone. Then, go outside and look around. Notice the setting. Are there trees and birds? Are there animals and parklands? Are there rocks and sand? Take in the scenery.

Then, using your camera, begin to take pictures of things that are interesting to you. Collect as many as you would like. When you return inside, download the pictures and print them on photo paper that you can turn into individual 4 × 6 or 5 × 7 cards to keep in your grounding kit.

The next time you want to reconnect with the present moment, take out your pack of nature cards and select one that resonates with you in that moment. Describe out loud what you see in the picture. The colors, the shapes, the objects. Are there animals? Plants? Rocks? Sky? What is it about this picture that was interesting to you? How do you feel when you look at the picture?

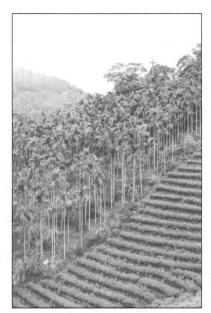
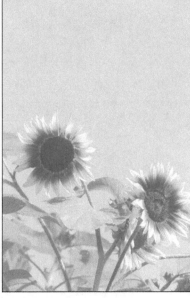
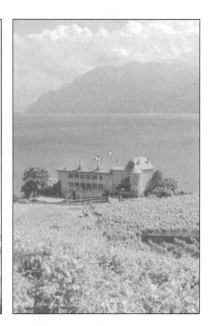

Hit the Ground

At times, trauma can make the body feel numb. This exercise will help you to reconnect with your body and ground your body to the present moment.

Find a space, either inside or outside, that is big enough for you to jump up and down without bumping into anyone or anything. Stand tall and stretch your arms to each side as far as you can, reaching in opposite directions. Then, bring them to your side. Next, inhale, lift your arms overhead, exhale, and JUMP. As you jump, forcefully bring your arms back to your sides. Again, inhale and lift your arms over your head, and exhale and JUMP, pushing your arms back down to your sides. Do this a couple of times until you feel present.

What did it feel like to move your body?

_____

_____

What felt more comfortable, arms up or down? Why?

_____

_____

Plug into Nature

Traumatic experiences affect the brain and body by keeping it in a constant state of hyperarousal. It is as if your body is constantly in "survival mode" and preparing itself for danger, even when there is no actual danger present. One way to quiet the body and calm the mind is to plug into nature. When you take in the sights that nature has to offer and listen to all of its sounds, this provides you with a naturally soothing experience.

For this exercise, find a digital device (e.g., phone, computer, tape recorder), that you can use to download nature sounds and videos. You can create these videos or soundtracks from a walk you have taken outdoors, or you can get them off the internet. If you type in "free nature soundtracks for download" into the search bar, you'll find many websites that have free videos and soundtracks you can use. Play around to see if there are certain sounds or scenes that you prefer or find more relaxing.

Once you have downloaded some options that work for you, you can play each video or soundtrack for 15 to 20 minutes whenever you feel the need to calm your body and quiet your mind. Listening to nature sounds is also a nice way to prepare for sleep.

As you listen to your nature downloads, notice how your body becomes more relaxed. If you have any anxious thoughts during this time, just make a note of that thought, put that thought on a cloud, and watch the cloud float away. Then, return to the soothing sounds and sights of nature.

Nature Drumsticks

It can be hard to talk about traumatic events. The words won't come, and the feelings can be so overwhelming that your body shuts down and becomes numb. Drumming is one form of expressive art that can help you communicate difficult stories and emotions. The rhythmic beat of the drum can connect you back to your body while also giving you a creative outlet to express yourself through music and sound. For this activity, you'll be using sandpaper and sticks you have gathered outside to create some nature drumsticks.

Go for a walk outside and collect two sticks that are approximately the same size and length. Try to find sticks that are sturdy and thick, and make sure they are a size that you would feel comfortable holding in your hands. Then, use sandpaper to smooth your sticks. Glide the sandpaper up and down the sides of your sticks, and notice how it feels to smooth the rough edges. Notice the shape that is forming with each rub of the sandpaper. It takes work, along with patience, to create the drumsticks.

Once you are satisfied with the preparation of your drumsticks, find a hard surface (e.g., rock, tree trunk, bench) and begin tapping the sticks on the surface. Notice how your hands feel tapping the sticks on the surfaces. Do you notice a beat? How do you feel when you beat fast? How do you feel when you beat slow?

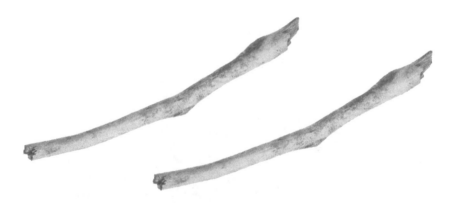

Group Fun:
Warriors

This activity is a group intervention that clinicians working with multiple children who have experienced trauma can use. It is a way to create a safe space for the healing of wounded warriors. It brings together children who have experienced trauma and can create a healing community.

Preparation
- Outdoor space with some wooded area
- Name tags
- Face paint
- Paintbrushes
- Sticks and stones for instruments

Instructions
1. Introduce this activity by gathering the children together and saying: *You are together because a terrible thing has happened to each of you. You are warriors on a similar path. The path is unpredictable and scary at times. However, by traveling together, you can share the burden. Warriors have long chosen names that identify their strength. Take a moment and think of your warrior name.*

2. Provide the children with name tags and markers that they can use to write down their warrior name. Have them wear the tag during this activity.

3. Then, prepare the children for the warrior ritual by helping them paint each other's faces. Encourage children to get creative as they put on their warrior paint.

4. Once the children are finished face painting, go outdoors and find a special place where you will hold the warrior ceremony. Once you find a space, claim it by creating a circle of safety. The circle can be made with string, rocks, sand, or sticks—anything that will create a physical boundary between the safe circle and the outside world.

5. When you are finished creating this sacred space, you may begin the ceremony. Sit in a circle and acknowledge that each of you are warriors. Introduce yourself with your warrior name that you have created.

6. When everyone has been introduced with their warrior name, have the children (as well as any co-therapists leading the activity) begin hitting sticks together or tapping stones together to create a united sound from the earth. This will solidify the warrior community.

7. When everyone has finished tapping (tap as long as you'd like), go around the circle and have each person identify their strength. After everyone has named their strength, ask each person to name something that they would like the group's help with. For example, maybe a child indicates that she is a really strong runner, but would like help with coping with bad thoughts or restless feelings. Specific answers to these help requests should not be given at this time. Rather, it is simply a chance for children to begin lowering the masks they have learned to wear to protect themselves following traumatic experiences. When everyone has had a turn, sit in silence acknowledging the warrior vow of solidarity.

8. Finish the ceremony by saying: *We sit here as warriors. We each possess strengths and things we need help with. Individually, these things may seem impossible, but with the strength of the group, we can help one another and lighten our burdens. We are warriors soldiering the path together.*

9. Lead the newly anointed warriors out of the sacred space and back to the gathering location, where you may have light refreshments to help transition from the group experience.

Nature Animation

Even though bad things can happen, sometimes amazing things can come out of it. Working through a difficult situation can sometimes result in positive learning or growth that strengthens the person, which is called *post-traumatic growth*. It is not unlike when a muscle is worked really hard, and miniscule tears may occur resulting in soreness or discomfort. However, when these tiny tears heal, the result is a stronger muscle.

This activity, which can be done in a small group format or with a single child, provides an opportunity for children to explore the path from devastation to recovery, and it offers a creative outlet for them to express feelings about their own difficult circumstances.

Find a device on which you can watch Igor Stravinsky's "The Firebird Suite," which is the final segment in Disney's *Fantasia 2000*. The animated movie clip is approximately 9 minutes long and set to the music of Stravinsky. It tells the story of a spring sprite and an elk who accidentally awaken the fury of a volcano (known as the "Firebird") that destroys the forest and, seemingly, the sprite. However, the sprite survives the ravaging flames of the volcano, and with the help of the elk, she restores the forest and brings all the plants back to life through her tears.

After you have watched the clip together, give children the opportunity to process what they have seen. For example, you might ask them to draw a picture about what they saw, or to journal about it. You can also ask them some prompting questions to gauge their understanding of the clip and its relevance to the notion of recovery and growth following trauma. For example, what is their understanding of what happened to the spring sprite? What did the elk do? Have they ever felt like this? Who helped them?

chapter
SEVEN

Mindfulness, Nature, and Grief Work with Children

Nicolas was just under 2 years of age when he attended his grandfather's funeral. He wandered through the sea of adults, holding tight to his mommy's and daddy's hands as he made his way to the front of the line where his grandfather lay peacefully in the casket. His grandmother picked him up as he tried to climb into the casket. "Sleeping?" he asked his grandmother. "No, sweetheart. Your grandfather died." Nicolas paused, looking at the man in the box and back at his grandmother. "Sleeping?" he tried again. "No, he has died. He is not sleeping," the grandmother replied softly. Nicolas looked around and attempted to contort his face mimicking the adults around him. "They are sad, honey. When someone dies, we can feel sad." His grandmother attempted to explain. Nicolas just watched, trying to imitate the adults around as the man in the box continued to sleep.

CHILDREN AND GRIEF

According to William Worden (2001), psychologist and grief expert, all children grieve regardless of age and stage of development. However, grief can be experienced in a variety of ways, and each stage of development provides a different manifestation or understanding of death and loss. For example, children may physically manifest grief in terms of somatic ailments, or they may experience it in terms of shock. They may feel anxious, angry, depressed, or withdrawn. They may act out behaviorally, resulting in biting or hitting. Additionally, there are critical periods of development where grief may impact the neurological development of a child in more significant ways. In this chapter, I'll examine the impact of grief on various stages of development and discuss how integrating the elements found in nature can aid in providing children with developmentally-appropriate support at each stage.

DEVELOPMENTAL GRIEF RESPONSES

Newborns and Toddlers

For newborns and toddlers, for whom object permanence is not established until approximately 28 months, grief may be experienced as annihilation of existence or a sense of abandonment. *Now, you see me, now you don't.* Loss at this age can result in a variety of challenges, including the desire to connect but not knowing how, a decrease in impulse control, uninhibited behavior (e.g., biting), and difficulty toilet training (DiCiacco, 2008). There may also be decreases in children's activity level (e.g., crawling, rolling over), decreases in appetite and possible weight loss, changes in sleep patterns, and increased irritability. Babies in particular may appear clingy and difficult to soothe.

Given that newborns and toddlers experience life through their senses, activities that promote sensory integration can support children of this age as they work through the bereavement process. As previously discussed, nature-informed activities represent one way to achieve sensory integration, as the subtle sensory stimuli afforded by nature is inherently soothing. For example, the natural lighting and soft sounds provided by an outdoor walk, or the soft touch of fur provided by a canine companion, can help newborns and toddlers to calm themselves and regulate their grief reactions. Similarly, the natural settings offer a variety of novel sensory stimuli (e.g., birds chirping, bright flowers, squirrels jumping from tree to tree, clouds floating across the sky) that attract the infant's attention and promote engagement in their surroundings.

Additionally, human-nature-animal connections provide a source of support and comfort for children, and simultaneously encourage interactive play. For example, the playful licks of a puppy or the movement of a goldfish in a bowl can provide infants and toddlers with gentle stimuli that contribute to interactive play. Children who have experienced separation from a parent and otherwise demonstrate a decreased interest in play may reach out to a family pet for comfort and soothing by nuzzling the animal. Promoting nondirected play at this age is crucial, as it allows children to symbolically "act out" feelings surrounding the loss that they would otherwise be unable to verbalize. In addition, the rolling and crawling that accompanies interactive play promotes vestibular development, which contributes to a calm and alert state, and soothes the hyperarousal from stress hormones likely experienced from the absence of a caretaker or loved one. "Through the play process, the infant also develops his or her unique conception of the environment as nurturing/ nonnurturing, safe/dangerous, and interesting/dull. In this manner, the infant begins to formulate a relationship to the external world of reality" (Nover, 1985, p. 22).

Early and Middle Childhood

As children continue in their development and begin to develop internal mental representations of their caregivers, they recognize attachment relationships and increasingly experience abandonment with loss. Children in early childhood (ages 2–6) do not fully understand the permanence of death and may believe that it is a temporary and reversible state. While they may be able to articulate that someone has passed away, the concept of what death means can still be a source of confusion. Some children may even experience magical thinking surrounding the topic, believing that they are somehow responsible for the other person's death.

As children progress into middle childhood (ages 6–10), they may become preoccupied with death, which may be demonized during this stage and personified in the form of a "boogeyman" or other monster. In addition, children can experience anxiety related to the idea of physical mutilation and may show concern about the experience of physical pain in death (DiCiacco, 2008). Questions such as, *does it hurt when you die? What happens when someone dies? What happens to the body? Do worms eat the body?* may become a focal point as children reach the end of this developmental stage and begin to better understand the permanence of death on the body.

Because children in this developmental stage may have difficulty fully articulating their feelings, grief can manifest in a variety of physical ways, including hyperactivity, emotional eating, and somatic complaints (DiCiacco, 2008). Children may withdraw, become argumentative and demanding, have difficulty concentrating, and exhibit a decrease in academic performance. Additionally, they may identify with the deceased and take on similar behaviors or symptoms that the deceased exhibited. For example, a 6-year-old boy may develop a somatic cough following the death of his grandfather who died of lung cancer.

In addition to the somatic and emotional expressions of grief during early childhood, children in middle childhood may experience social pressures around grieving. Children in this stage are beginning to develop a greater awareness of the impact of their peer relationships. The belief that everyone is watching them (e.g., the "imaginary audience") may inform the grief process by adding internal judgment around the child's mourning. Beliefs such as, *I should be sad, but I am not. I am angry!* or *I have to be strong for my family* may affect the child's expectations around the grief process.

To process through their loss, there are a variety of ways that children in early and middle childhood can benefit from interacting with the natural settings. Not only do the natural settings provide a source of sensory integration and social connectedness, but they also provide a means by which children can examine the cycle of life and death. By middle childhood, children may have already experienced the death of a pet or plant, and they have begun crafting a schema about life and death. Birds are hatched from eggs and fed by their parents. When baby birds are ready to test their wings, they leap from the safety of their nest to fly. At times, these maiden voyages fail, and the babies fall from the safety of the branches and die. As children witness this cycle of life in nature, it provides them with a framework from which they can further craft their understanding regarding death and dying. Similarly, as burial rituals are understood at this age, shoeboxes can become caskets in which children lovingly place a newly deceased animal (e.g., bird, frog, hamster) to rest and return it to its home in nature.

Adolescents

Adolescents are capable of abstract thinking and struggle with the concepts of being versus nonbeing. While teens may feel immortal, they have an increased understanding of death and permanence, resulting in increased death anxiety. Teens may have experienced a variety of losses at this point and can differentiate between different types of losses. For example, in addition to pets and plants, adolescents may have experienced the loss of family members, such as grandparents or great aunts and uncles. Additionally, they may have experienced more disenfranchised loss from such events as changing schools, moving to a different neighborhood, broken friendships, romantic heartbreaks, and physical illness. For others, it may be their first experience with loss.

Grief may manifest in a variety of ways in adolescence, including unpredictable emotional bursts, academic difficulties, and trouble sleeping, eating, and concentrating. The loss of a sibling, peer, or parent may also elicit survivor's guilt, causing teens to question why they are still alive. Teens may self-medicate and exhibit increased risk-taking behavior (e.g., drinking, drugs, reckless driving, promiscuous sex) as a means of testing out their own mortality or escaping intense feelings. They may also manifest the loss by acting out or withdrawing socially (DiCiacco, 2008). *Thanatechnology*, or the use of media and technology during the mourning process, is commonly used by teens to express their "virtual" grief and may provide a source of comfort and connection. However, the use of social media during this vulnerable time may also be used to glamorize loss in an unhealthy manner.

Spending time in nature, particularly in untamed natural environments, has been shown to provide therapeutic support to teenagers as they navigate through and process their loss (Combs, Hoag, Javorski, & Roberts, 2016). Wilderness therapy allows teens (and all the hormones raging through their bodies) to surge through the unpaved, untrimmed, and unsculptured environment and come face-to-face with the drama found in nature. They can witness the snake eating the bird along the pine needle trail. They can sprawl the rocky edge of a hill to reach the peak overlook and see the eagles soaring below. They can ride the rapids of a fast-flowing river and be plunged (breathless) into the stillness of a stream and float in silence to shore. While not necessary, these wildlife experiences offer teens the opportunity to face their fears and cheat death by connecting with the elements and mastering the terrain.

DISENFRANCHISED GRIEF

At times, children's experiences of grief are dismissed as unimportant or irrelevant. For example, the death of a beloved pet, parental separation, or a move to another school district are all examples of situations that may provide a significant sense of loss for a child. Chronic illness or trauma are other examples associated with tremendous loss that are often overlooked or minimized. For those of us working with children, it is important to recognize these losses and validate the experience of grief so that children can receive the necessary support during this difficult time. If we are not sufficiently attuned to the extent of a child's grief, then we may overlook certain emotional and behavioral cues associated with the loss, and misinterpret or needlessly pathologize a child's symptoms.

Even the most well-intentioned clinician or educator may misread and pathologize a child's lack of concentration, fidgeting, and restless behavior. Indeed, this was the case for 5½-year-old Andrew, whose dog, Ranger, died suddenly from a heart attack. Andrew was very close to Ranger, and even though his parents provided him with age-appropriate information around the death, Andrew began eliciting restless and inattentive behavior at school. His teacher, aware of the death, still sent notes home daily indicating that Andrew was disruptive in class. On the last day of the week, the teacher's note read, "Andrew is exhibiting signs of ADHD," despite the fact that Andrew had not previously exhibited any difficulties in class. This example is one of misdiagnosis. Andrew did not need medication or treatment for ADHD; he was simply grieving and needed support. He was trying to figure out the concept of death against his understanding of his love for his dog.

FOUR STAGES OF GRIEF WORK

Children are incredibly resilient and fluid in their grief. At times, it may resemble a roller coaster ride of varied emotion. For example, I once worked with a distraught young widow who brought her 7-year-old daughter to see me because she thought her daughter was repressing her feelings over the recent and sudden death of her father. "She will become tearful in the morning and ask about her father, then run off to play with her friends as if everything is status quo. I just want to be sure that she is alright." This young child was, in fact, attending to her grief in a healthy manner. She allowed herself to miss her father and then resumed her normally scheduled routine. The ebb and flow of her grief allowed her to manage her day-to-day activities.

According to psychologist and grief expert, William Worden (2001), children experience grief through a series of nonlinear tasks. One of the first tasks in mourning is to *recognize the reality of the loss*. As previously indicated, depending on a child's stage of development, a child may experience this differently. For example, 3-year-old Tara may wait at the door for her mother to return from "death" as if she is on a business trip, while 13-year-old Tom keeps listening to the last message his father left on his cell phone. The process of realizing the permanency of the loss may take time and effort as children navigate (as they are able) the emotional pain and the day-to-day changes that accompany the loss. Participating in death rituals (e.g., funerals and memorial services) can help children in moving toward this realization, as can engaging in the comfort of natural settings that offer examples of the normalcy of the life-death cycle.

The second task in mourning is to *work through the pain of the loss.* As previously discussed, grief and loss can be expressed in a variety of ways. The infant may withdraw from play. The young child may begin wetting the bed. The adolescent may start skipping classes or experiment with substances. It is important for caregivers and educators to promote healthy grief expression (e.g., journaling, expressive arts, counseling) while monitoring for unhealthy behaviors. Nature and animal-assisted engagement is one way to promote soothing comfort and symbolic emotional expression.

The third task in mourning includes *adjusting to the environment in which the deceased is missing.* A variety of secondary losses may occur as a result of the primary loss. For example, changes in living situations may occur, like moving to a more affordable home or with relatives. Expectations around household chores may also change. In the case of pet loss, there need to be decisions made about what to do with the pet bowls, leashes, bedding, and toys that have been integrated into the family home. Following the death of our beloved Goldendoodle puppy, Lily, we discussed what the family members wanted to do with Lily's toys and bed. Some members wanted to keep the items where they had always been (sometimes underfoot), while others wanted them put away because it was too overwhelming to view the items without Lily. Candid and frequent communication can help children navigate this difficult task.

The ultimate and final task of grief work is to *"emotionally relocate" the loss in a way that allows the child to move forward* (Worden, 2001). That is, it involves helping children discover healthy ways to stay emotionally connected to the deceased while, at the same time, helping them understand that life will (and does) go on. This goal can be accomplished by helping children find ways to memorialize their loved one, while also allowing themselves to form new relationships that in no way replace the person whom they've lost. As the following case study illustrates, the natural world offers a holistic venue for grief work that helps children maintain an enduring connection with what they have lost, while also allowing them to form a new connection to something that provides a sense of awe, wonder, and hope.

Case Study

TARA

Tara, a 14-year-old girl, presented to therapy with grief related to the tragic death of her friend. The classmate had ultimately succumbed following a lengthy battle with leukemia. The classmate's parents involved her friends in the memorial service, and the school had sponsored a rally to raise funds for a national organization in her honor. However, these rituals and memorials just didn't feel like they were enough to grieving Tara. One afternoon, while sitting on the picnic bench near my office, Tara proclaimed that she wanted to do something special for her friend. Something that would help her feel connected and could be shared by others. Tara and her friend loved to watch the butterflies in the fields. Tara even suggested that this was the way her friend communicated with her—as a butterfly.

With little prompting, Tara decided to plant a butterfly garden in her friend's honor near a common teen hang out. She recruited her parents to help her get permission to create this garden on the commercial property and to finance some of the plants. Tara spent several weekends diligently researching plants, designing plans, selecting plants, and digging up the space to host the new garden. When she was finished, she took pictures and brought them to session. It was truly beautiful. What a legacy to her dear friend, and now, every time Tara and her friends gathered, they could be in the presence of their classmate through the fluttering of the beautiful butterflies.

SUMMARY AND EXERCISES

Children's experience of grief and loss is physical, emotional, and spiritual. By engaging with nature, children can find creative and meaningful ways to reconnect with that which they have lost. It also provides them with a plethora of opportunities to witness the cycle of life. The rhythm of the tides, the changing of the seasons, and the rise and fall of the sun and moon offer moments to explore the natural progression of life and death, of beginnings and endings. The rhythm of the natural world is consistent and predictable, which provides comfort in its fidelity to even the youngest bereaved.

The pages that follow include a variety of nature-based mindfulness activities that promote the candid exploration of death and loss. The first handout provides caregivers and educators with a brief summary of the symptoms related to children's grief and explains how engaging in nature can ease these symptoms and promote deeper healing. **The worksheets and handouts that follow contain activities that are intended to help children examine death and loss, and promote creative expression and meaning construction in the grief process.**

Mindfulness, Nature, and Grief Work with Children

All children experience grief, regardless of age. However, each stage of development offers diverse ways in which grief may be experienced. For example, newborns and toddlers are still struggling with the realization that just because an object is not visible does not mean it has disappeared. Therefore, parental separation, relocation, or death may be experienced as banishment.

However, as children continue to develop, they will experience a variety of losses over time and begin to realize the permanence of loss. This may cause them to experience death anxiety and increased fears about the safety of themselves or others. In addition, the experience of grief does not only pertain to issues surrounding death and loss, as chronic illness and traumatic events are often accompanied by grief as well.

This grief can manifest in a variety of physical, emotional, and behavioral ways.

Physical	Emotional	Behavioral
• Shock	• Fear	• Acting out
• Dizziness	• Anxiety	• Regressive behavior (e.g., bedwetting, incontinence)
• Somatic complaints (e.g., aches and pains)	• Anger	• Social withdrawal
	• Shame and guilt	• Risk-taking behavior
	• Depression	
	• Indifference and despair	

Engaging in the natural surroundings is one way to promote resiliency and coping among grieving children, as the experiences offered by nature promote a calm and alert state, and they facilitate sensory integration versus sensory overload.

In addition, interacting with nature further encourages creative expression and meaning-making around the difficult and often abstract concept of death and loss. By witnessing the natural cycle of life and the changing of the four seasons, children can develop a framework for understanding concepts of life and death, and of beginnings and endings.

Nature's stories of birds, bees, and butterflies offer a matter-of-fact exploration of loss that can be soothing and restorative at any age.

My Rock Tale

Sometimes it is hard to talk about our losses. We may feel shy or just want our story to be private. However, telling our stories is important, even if we just tell it to ourselves. This activity allows you to tell your story of loss through the creative expression of rocks.

Imagine that rocks could tell your story by their shapes, sizes, colors, or weight. What type of rock would represent how you are feeling right now? Go for a walk and look for rocks that best depict your current story. Is your rock smooth and shiny, or is it chipped or jagged in certain areas? Does it have layers of color? Is your rock solo or is it in a pile? Choose a rock that best depicts your current life story, and then use the following spaces to have the rock "tell" your life story.

Once upon a time, there was a rock…

_____

_____

_____

_____

_____

_____

_____

_____

_____

_____

_____

_____

_____

_____

The Shadow Knows

There are many sides to us. Sometimes we are happy. Other times we are sad. Nature has different sides as well. There is daytime and nighttime. There is light and dark. Living things that are born will one day die. Looking at the dark side of things can be helpful in showing us what may be hidden in the shadows of our own thoughts and emotions.

Preparation

- White drawing paper
- Black crayon, colored pencil, or marker
- Gold or bright yellow crayon, colored pencil, or marker

Instructions

1. On a bright sunny day, go outside and find an area where shadows are being cast. Choose a shadow that interests you and examine it. What is in it or on it? What is its shape?

2. Draw or trace the shadow on your drawing paper, and shade in all the dark shadow areas with your black marker or crayon. Then, give the shadow a name.

3. Give the shadow a voice by writing a conversation between you and the shadow.

4. Use your gold or yellow crayon to fill in the white spaces created between the black shadow areas of your drawing. Notice the beautiful lightness against the dark and how they coexist in nature—and in you.

5. Reflect on this activity by answering the questions on the reflection worksheet.

Adapted from Sweeney (2013)

The Shadow Knows Reflection

What did you name the shadow? Why did you choose this name?

_____

_____

_____

Did the shadow have a name for you? What was it?

_____

_____

_____

What did you and the shadow talk about?

_____

_____

_____

What was it like to talk to the shadow?

_____

_____

_____

Dams and Leaks

Loss is accompanied by many emotions. It is important to take the time to observe and release these emotions so they don't continue to build up inside of us over time. Just like flowing water, our emotions can get "dammed up" (stuck) and then burst out in other ways. While our emotions and thoughts are not all of us, they are part of us. This activity will help you explore some of the feelings you are having right now around your loss so you can identify ways to keep the "water" flowing.

Go for a walk by a stream or river, or watch the flow of water on a digital device or tabletop stream. Watch how the water can get stuck over time by the buildup of rocks, sticks, and debris. When the stream becomes stopped, the pressure builds and overflows—at times in harmful ways. The same can happen with our emotions if we don't provide different outlets for the river to flow.

Identify some outlets for your emotions (your "water") to keep it flowing in a healthy manner. For example, running and jumping can release emotions. Drawing and painting can help emotions flow across a page. Writing can capture the feelings that you are experiencing. Put those words to music and create a song. All of these are great ways to let your emotions flow. Can you think of other ways to keep a healthy flow of emotions?

Adapted from Chown (2018)

Keepsake Nest

A nest is a small structure that animals create to provide shelter and comfort for their families. You've probably seen bird nests before, but there are several other animals that build nests too, including fish, turtles, insects, rabbits, and squirrels. In this activity, you'll be creating your own keepsake nest to store important or meaningful letters, pictures, or gifts that remind you of a loved one who has passed away. One of the most important ways that we stay connected to those we have lost is to gather items that remind us of them. Create a nest using a variety of possible items, and decorate it to make it special.

Preparation

- Item to use as a "nest" (e.g., paper bag, wooden box, basket)
- Craft items (e.g., glitter, yarn, glue, scissors, feathers, ribbon)

Instructions

1. Find a space where you can work outdoors and spread out the craft items that you would like to use to decorate your nest.

2. Spend some time decorating the outside of your nest to make it look special. Maybe you want to sprinkle it with different colors of glitter, or maybe you want to glue a bunch of feathers to the side of it. The choice is yours.

3. After you are done decorating your nest, find some items that you would like to include in the nest that remind you of your loved one. These items can include cards, letters, jewelry, pictures, or—for a pet—an old collar. It can be anything that reminds you of the person or pet you have lost.

4. Place these items in your nest and arrange them in any way that you choose. Spend some time looking through the items and reminiscing about the times you and your loved one had together.

5. Put your keepsake nest somewhere safe, and open it up whenever you want to look back and remember your loved one.

6. Answer the reflection questions on the reflection worksheet.

Keepsake Nest Reflection

How did you decide to make your nest?

_____

_____

_____

What items did you choose to keep in the nest? Why?

_____

_____

_____

What do you feel when you are looking at the items in the nest? Sometimes we have more than one feeling.

_____

_____

_____

Fire Bowl Ritual

Grief is a time of letting go and holding on at the same time. We can let go of the physical aspects of a loved one, a toxic relationship, or familiar schoolyard friends while holding on to cherished memories, lessons learned, and foundational friendships, respectively. This activity allows children to reflect on what they are letting go of and holding on to in the midst of their grief work, including the additional loss they may experience when counseling sessions end. It taps into the creative and meaningful reflection often accompanied by loss.

Preparation

- Fire bowl, fireplace, or firepit
- Slips of paper
- 2- to 3-inch stones
- Permanent marker
- Matches or lighter
- Pot holder

Instructions

1. Ask the child to write something down on the slip of paper that they would like to leave behind after your time together ends. It may be a feeling such as *anger* at their loved one for dying. It could be *sadness* about the counseling sessions ending, as this can also be experienced as a loss. It is something that the child no longer wants to hold on to regarding the death of the loved one, or the grief around ending counseling.

2. Ask them to write something down on the stone that they would like to take with them and remember from your time together. It could be something that they discovered about themselves or a memory of their time with you or their deceased loved one.

3. After the child has finished writing, ask them to place the rock and the paper in the fire bowl. They may want to say something like a favorite memory (of their loved one or of their time with you in counseling), a poem, or prayer.

4. Light the fire bowl and sit with the child as they watch the fire release what they want to leave behind and solidify what they want to keep.

5. Wait until the fire settles and the stone cools, and use a pot holder to safely remove the stone from the fire bowl. Give the stone to the child as a keepsake and transitional object for this memory.

Borrowed with permission from Susan Coale,
Director of Hospice of the Chesapeake's Family Life Center

Group Fun:
Family Portrait I

You can use this group exercise with children who are experiencing not only a family death, but with those who are experiencing parental separation, divorce, or deployment of family members as well. It allows children to recreate family memories and reconnect with their loved one through expressive means of drawing and role-playing.

Preparation
- Paper
- Crayons or colored pencils
- Glue
- Scissors
- Space to recreate a family memory

Instructions
1. Have each child in the group think of their favorite family memory. It could be a holiday they shared with the loved one they are missing or a family vacation—a time that they cherish.

2. Have the children draw the memory using whatever creative means they want. They can color, paint, or use markers. They may want to glue glitter or beads. Encourage them to be as expressive as they want to be.

3. Tell the children that they are going to be the director of their memory. They need to provide the other members in the group with instructions as to how to "act out" the family memory. Decide which group members are going to pretend to be which family members, and then have the child direct the memory.

4. After the group has finished enacting the memory, talk about the experience and help children reflect on the activity with some of the following questions:

   - Who is in your memory?

   - What are you doing in your memory?

   - What was it like to remember?

   - What was it like to see other people acting out your memory?

   - What do you miss most about your loved one?

   - What thoughts make you happy? Sad?

Family Portrait II

This activity can be done in either an individual or group format, and it allows children to recreate family connections by viewing the connections found in animal or insect homes. Children will be able to examine family roles and structure in a creative manner by exploring their own family dynamics through the lens of animal or insect families.

Preparation
- Outdoor setting that offers a variety of habitats (e.g., trees, flowers, bushes, nests)

Instructions
1. Take a walk outside with the child or group of children, and look for any animal or insect homes that you come across. These homes may be found in flowers or plants, or in nests and hives.

2. While viewing animal or insect homes, have children describe the family connections that they see. Ask them to describe how each member in the animal or insect home has a role in the family, and have them relate this to their own family dynamics.

   - Is there a parental role in the animal or insect home? Or does everyone take care of each other?

   - Who is the caregiver in the child's home? What is the child's role in the family? Is the child the oldest? The youngest?

   - How many members belong to the animal or insect home?

   - How many members live in the child's home?

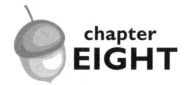

chapter
EIGHT

Nature-Based Mindfulness for Empathy and Value Development

> *"You can judge a man's true character by the way he treats his fellow animals."*
>
> — Paul McCartney

VALUE DEVELOPMENT AND EMPATHY

Children begin to develop a moral understanding of what is right and wrong beginning at an early age. For example, 3-year-old Melinda may see Carl take some toy blocks out of Kevin's hands and say, "Carl! You're gonna get in trouble!" Kevin's tears resulting from the removal of his blocks may prompt Carl to return the blocks, or Melinda may bring other toys to Kevin to ease his pain. These experiences, in turn, help children learn how to understand and share in the feelings and motives of others, which promotes the development of empathy and value-laden behavior.

One way to facilitate the development of empathy and values in childhood is to provide ample opportunities for human-animal and human-nature interactions. Interacting with animals and plants provides a mutual exchange of behavior that allows children to view the impact of their own behaviors on the environment (Hyde, 2008; Kahn & Kellert, 2002). Through these interactions, children learn how to be attuned to subtle cues provided by animals and plants. If the child waters the plant, then it remains green and lush. If the child forgets to water the plant, then it shrivels and dies. If the child is too loud, then the animal may cower and hide. If the child uses a gentle touch, then the animal may move toward the child to receive more interaction.

There exists rich data demonstrating that even children with autism spectrum disorder—who have profound difficulties in identifying and responding to social cues—can benefit from this connection with nature in promoting the development of empathy and social understanding (Abreu & Figueiredo, 2015; Beetz, 2017; Dawson, 2016; Dunlop & Tsantefski, 2017). For example, at the therapeutic ranch Eye of a Horse, teenagers diagnosed with autism are invited to slowly walk into a field of cows and watch how the cows respond to their presence. If the teens walk quickly toward the cows, then the cows rush away. If the teens stand still, allowing the cows to get accustomed to their presence, then the cows slowly return to their grazing pattern, undisturbed by the teens watching them. Through this program, teens are soon able to describe the behavior of the cows based on this new perspective and, more importantly, bridge the behavior of the cows to human behavior (e.g., other people may run away if they are approached too quickly, but they may feel more comfortable if approached in a more relaxed and gradual manner).

Simply put, the natural elements provide children with the experiences needed to develop the capacity for empathy and construct a set of values associated with ethical, prosocial, and compassionate behavior. In this chapter, I'll discuss the human-nature-animal connection in greater detail, specifically with regard to its impact on spiritual, value, and character development.

NATURE, EMPATHY, AND BONDING

Those of us who have pets understand the tremendous complexity of the human-animal connection. The love is deep and the loss great. When we connect with others, including animals, our body releases a potent hormone and neurotransmitter called oxytocin. This biochemical is released during intimate moments, such as when mothers nurse their newborn babies and when we experience romantic intimacy with our partners. It is a strong bonding agent, so to speak. What is even more fascinating is that during human-animal interaction, not only is oxytocin released in the human, but it is also released in the animal! (Olmert, 2009).

Unfortunately, oxytocin has an approximate 20-minute shelf life and requires continuous administration to maintain its effects. However, additional exposure to bonding experiences can cultivate oxytocin receptor cells in the body, which may facilitate more frequent and positive experiences of social interactions. Oxytocin is associated with greater trust and prosocial behavior in the context of interpersonal interactions (Kosfeld et al., 2005). These findings have implications for interventions for children with autism, who have been found to exhibit low levels of oxytocin, as well as variations in oxytocin receptor cells, compared to neurotypical children. In particular, increased oxytocin receptor cells may contribute to greater opportunities for children with autism to recognize and respond with socially-appropriate cues, in turn contributing to the development of empathy. Research has found that intranasal inhalation of oxytocin improves social skills among children with autism, particularly among those with the lowest baseline levels of oxytocin prior to treatment (Parker et al., 2017). Therefore, oxytocin administration appears to be promising in the treatment of children with autism spectrum disorder.

SPIRITUALITY AND EMPATHY

Spiritual awareness appears to underpin altruistic and ethical behavior, as it provides a framework regarding what is right versus what is wrong. Spirituality also provides a lens to examine existential questions surrounding value and meaning, which informs our worldview and how we make meaning out of our circumstances (Andrews & Marotta, 2005; Hyde, 2008; Pargament, 2011). It also provides us with a sense of embodied well-being and connectedness to something bigger. For example, 5-year-old Eric found comfort in understanding that his recently deceased grandmother was now in heaven playing with her dog, Callie, who had died two years before.

According to Hyde (2008), there are four characteristics of children's spirituality. First, it involves an embodied experience in that children experience spirituality through their senses. Hyde describes this as a *felt sense*, an awareness of *flow*, or being so captivated and in harmony that it is fully encompassing. For children, spirituality is experienced through the integration of all the sensory organs in the here-and-now. For example, Hyde (2008) recounts the experience of 5-year-old Cindy:

Once, when I was lining up at the end of lunch time, I was looking at a bird on the ground not far from me. I think it was a sparrow, because it was really little. The teacher must have called for us to walk into class, but I was still looking at the bird. My back was turned away from the teacher and I didn't realize that my line had moved, and suddenly I was standing by myself.
(p. 85)

In this manner, Cindy experienced the bird in the moment with all of her senses. She experienced a conscious awareness that led her to reflect on something bigger than (and beyond) herself and that involved a recognition of a much more collective self. Providing children with opportunities to connect with other living beings and natural settings promotes this experience of embodied conscious awareness. Just like Cindy was able to get lost in just *being* with the sparrow, children can experience the world with greater awareness and higher consciousness that promotes empathy and altruism as they recognize themselves as part of a bigger picture.

Second, spirituality in childhood involves an integrated awareness in that children are able to see the interconnectedness between humans, animals, and nature. Essentially, children recognize on some level that they belong to a bigger picture as they connect with living creatures and the natural world, and this realization of connectedness cultivates the development of empathy. For example, children tasked with building a fort will navigate the collection of resources, the strategy of construction, and the physicality of building all the while attending to the needs of the builders. Children will recognize that this is a team effort, and even young children will ultimately move in the direction of cooperation and unified action. This process extends beyond cooperative play and reflects an emerging higher level of conscious awareness not only of the task at hand, but also of the relationships of the other children involved. It ultimately reflects an understanding (albeit less sophisticated) of universality and unity.

Third, for children, spirituality is woven with a variety of meaning threads. That is, children express their spirituality and meaning-making around the ultimate questions of death, life, and suffering through a variety of ideas and concepts that help them create a personal framework regarding these issues. Because children experience the world in a variety of ways, it allows them to accept more than one way of viewing the world. When asked the question, "What do you think happens after we die?" children may provide diverse answers that resemble a blend of dogma. For example, 6-year-old Katie stated that her dog, Sadie, was now in heaven with Jesus and her grandmother (reflecting a Christian perspective). However, Katie also noted that her neighbor's dog had just given birth to puppies, so perhaps Sadie was one of the puppies (reflecting a belief in reincarnation). Encouraging respectful discussion of children's worldviews and promoting acceptance of a variety of perspectives promotes an atmosphere of empathy, altruism, and acceptance.

Finally, spirituality in childhood involves constant searching as children naturally seek out novel experiences. Children are little scientists and theologians, looking for meaning (and spiders) under rocks and in bushes. They naturally seek out what inspires awe and wonder, and they become quietly reflective when offered the opportunity. For example, my Floridian grandson had never experienced snow until during an early December trip when he visited with me in Maryland. We were walking my dog when the snowflakes began to flutter toward the ground. He suddenly put up his hand to halt the walk. "Yaya [the name he calls me], what is that?" he whispered. "It is a snowflake," I confirmed. His eyes grew wide and he plunged his tongue into the air attempting to catch the elusive frozen drops. He began to twirl with delight as the snowfall grew heavy and began to stick on his gloves, as well as his tongue. In complete silence, we twirled and caught snowflakes. He experienced snow for the first time with awe and wonder—and a quiet reverence.

Therefore, for children, spirituality is experienced through the senses, promotes interrelatedness, and offers inspirational reflection, in addition to beauty and wonder. When allowed to continue their quest, children will experience the world as novel, inspiring, and interconnected. It becomes a world that they don't simply live in, but that they belong to and hold accountability for. Others matter—animals matter, the earth matters, and they begin to craft a way to keep it that way.

As clinicians and educators, we can promote empathy and value development in children by offering opportunities for whole-body experiences that provide awe and wonder, and that create moments of reflection around the ultimate and existential questions of humanity. Engaging with the natural environment and its creatures provides this very environment, as it fosters the development of a psychospiritual framework that promotes value and character development, and a greater sense of empathy for all creation.

Nature, Spirituality, and Value Development

Eco-spirituality describes the connection between humans and the natural environment in the context of interrelatedness and the sacred. Eco-spirituality promotes spiritual, value, and character development by recognizing the many opportunities to examine the separateness and interrelatedness inherent in human-animal-nature interactions. From a very early age, we are attracted to what is novel and appealing, and through our interactions, we learn to interact with the natural element. Wasps sting, birds fly, and snakes slither. We begin to connect to the natural world and learn about the "other" and how to commune with the "other." It is beautiful to witness children interacting in the natural world. It is inspiring and sacred. For example,

Eight-year-old Miranda is at the seashore with her father Mark. She wades out into the shallow water and stands there, the water coming up to her waist. She begins to move back and forth with the waves. Ten or fifteen minutes pass. Mark manages to sit and simply watch, not interrupting. He finds his body swaying with Miranda's. Still, he does not interrupt, despite his fears that she might be having some kind of seizure, or whether she has enough sunscreen on. After a long while Miranda turns and comes out of the water, absolutely glowing and peaceful, Mark later said. She sits down next to her father. After a few minutes, he gently asks what she has been doing. "I was the water," she says softly. "The water?" he repeats. "Yeah, it was amazing. I was the water. I love it and it loves me. I don't know how else to say it." They sit quietly until a few minutes later she hops up to dig in the sand. "Somehow I felt completely overwhelmed, like I had witnessed grace," Mark said later. (Hart, 2003, p. 47)

Miranda experienced a connectedness to the water that was awe-inspiring and sacred. She gained a greater understanding of the beauty and wonder of the ocean. That experience is forever a part of her eco-spiritual framework that will inform her interactions with the ocean.

In addition to the significant connectedness, children's eco-spirituality and its connection to nature poses ethical considerations. What happens if I step on the worm? Or put salt on a slug? How does throwing plastic in the water affect the fish and sea life? How does impacting the environment affect humans? What is my role in taking care of the earth? The ability to struggle with these questions cultivates an understanding of interconnectedness among humans, animals, and the earth that promotes empathy toward all living creatures. We are separate but interrelated. The wellness of one species informs the wellness of all species.

SUMMARY AND EXERCISES

Direct engagement in nature provides opportunities to cultivate empathy and a value-laden framework that translates into pro-social, empathetic, and caring behavior. We can help children in this process of empathy development by providing opportunities for human-animal and human-nature interactions. After all, in the words of philosopher Thomas Berry, "The universe is composed of subjects to be communed with, not objects to be exploited. Everything has its own voice. [...] and they constitute a community of existence that is profoundly related."

The pages that follow include a variety of nature-based mindfulness activities that promote the development of empathy, values, and spiritual awareness. The first handout provides caregivers and educators with a brief summary describing children's spirituality and the role it plays in developing empathy and values. The worksheets and handouts that follow contain activities that are intended to help children cultivate empathy by creating a sense of interrelatedness to nature, animals, and all living creatures.

Nature-Based Mindfulness for Empathy and Value Development

Children begin to develop concepts of what is appropriate and inappropriate behavior from birth. Value development and empathy are essential in social interaction and satisfactory communion with others. Empathy, or the ability to understand and share the feelings or experiences of another, is a critical element in establishing and maintaining relationships.

Children's ability to understand another's experience is related to developmental stage, neurological makeup, and experiences. Activities that promote interacting with one another encourage the release of oxytocin, a hormone and neurotransmitter that is present in bonding experiences.

Importantly, spirituality underpins altruistic and ethical behavior, as it informs our worldview and meaning-making, and it provides a framework for existential questions surrounding value and meaning. Spirituality is experienced as a sense of embodied well-being and connectedness to something bigger, and it can include explicit or intrinsic spirituality. Explicit spirituality includes rituals, sacred texts, and stories of specific faith communities. Intrinsic spirituality refers to those activities that promote awe and wonder and inspire reflection on the existential questions around life, death, suffering, and purpose.

We can promote empathy and value development in children by offering opportunities that are whole-body and that inspire quiet reflection, awe, and wonder. Interacting directly with nature and animals provides just the environment!

Flower Power

All living creatures need food, water, shelter, and kindness. Plants and flowers need to be provided with the right amount of sunshine, water, and plant food to grow strong and healthy. Additionally, sprinkling in a few kind words such as, "You can do it! You are strong!" or "What beautiful petals you have today!" can even encourage a tiny seedling.

Preparation

- A container to grow seeds
- Potting soil
- Seeds
- Water spritzer bottle
- Plant care journal to log your daily interactions with the seed (and eventual plant)

Instructions

1. Find a container that you would like to use to grow your seed. This could be a paper cup, an empty egg container, or a pretty ceramic pot.

2. Place the soil in the container you have decided to use to grow the seed.

3. Decide what seeds you want to plant. Do you want flowers, such as daisies or sunflowers? Or do you want to grow vegetables, such as tomatoes or squash? Or perhaps you like the smell of herbs, such as lavender or rosemary? All of these plants produce flowers, for a season. Perhaps you would like to plant them all and create a garden. It doesn't matter. You decide what you want to plant and provide care for.

4. Plant the seed in the container, and place the container near a window where it will get plenty of sunshine.

5. Water the seed just a little bit with the spritzer bottle every couple of days to keep the soil moist but not too wet.

6. Communicate with the plant in a kind way. Encourage it to grow big and strong.

7. As you are able, keep a journal each day about the care and growth of the plant. As you write in your journal, what do you observe as you take care of the seed? What does the plant need to be healthy? What ways do you show kindness toward the plant? How is this the same and different from caring for a friend?

Be Like a Flower

Being teased is no fun! No one likes to be bullied. So, what should you do? One way to help yourself in this situation is to use your mindful breathing skills. Instead of getting angry with the other person, just look at them, breathe deeply, and smile like a flower. Flowers just smile, regardless of the weather. You, too, can breathe deeply, smile, and hold compassion for the other person who is clearly not happy, which is why they are trying to make other people unhappy. The next time that someone tries to bully you or tease you, return to your breath and tell yourself the following:

Breathing in, I feel calm.

Breathing out, I am not going to get angry.

Breathing in, I am fresh as a flower.

Breathing out, I am solid as a mountain.

However, being calm and breathing mindfully doesn't mean that you shouldn't take care of yourself. If someone is making you feel scared or unsafe, then you need to take the necessary steps to protect yourself. Make sure to go to a safe space and ask a trusted adult for help.

Adapted from Hanh (2011)

Friends Without Fur

Having a pet helps us learn how to care for someone (or something) other than ourselves. When we are able to care for others and see their perspective, we are *empathizing* with them. Empathy means that we can understand how they feel and share in their experience. For example, when my dog sits in front of me with his ball, I know he wants to play fetch. When he stands in front of the door and makes a whiny noise, I know he needs to go outside and go to the bathroom—or chase a squirrel. When a cat curls up and begins to purr softly, that means she is very happy. While having a cat or dog may be fun, not everyone is able to have one. Here are some other friendly creatures to connect with:

- **Betta:** Fish are great to watch and are relatively manageable. Bettas live alone and can be wonderful to provide care for as they live in small containers, enjoy some distraction and interaction, and demand very little.
- **Birds:** Birds provide endless entertainment. They can be messy, though. So be certain that you learn how to care for them before you invest in one.
- **Carnivorous plant:** Buy a Venus flytrap or other plant that eats bugs. Spend time learning about how to care for the plant. Be certain that it has the right amount of sun, shade, water, and bugs!

If owning a friend without fur is not possible, how about adopting a natural element? Here are some other ideas:

- **Local birds:** Hang a bird feeder near a window and watch as your local winged neighbors come to visit each day. Use your journal to write down the different types of birds you see over the season. Remember to keep the feeder filled with yummy seeds.
- **Bees:** Hosting a honey beehive is a lot of work, but it's very rewarding. If you want to help these pollinators with a bit less stress, you can make or purchase a Mason bee house. Here is a link for an easy bee home: https://www.turningclockback.com/diy-mason-bee-house.
- **Butterflies:** Helping butterflies involves very little effort. Find out what your favorite butterfly eats, and grow it in your garden. I love monarch butterflies, so I plant lots of milkweed in my yard.
- **Bats:** Bats are great visitors. They help keep pesky bugs out of the yard. Hang a bat house high in a tree or on a shed in your yard and wait until dark to watch your new friends hard at work.
- **Plant or tree:** Take special care of a plant or tree in your yard. Spend time learning what helps it grow and stay strong. Watch how it changes over the seasons.
- **River or lake:** Is there a river, creek, or lake nearby? Commit to spending time keeping it litter-free. Watch the changes that occur over the seasons.
- **Star:** Spend time getting to know a particular star in the sky. Watch how it moves over the seasons.

A Question for Nature

As with all relationships, connecting with nature can be interactive and supportive. Nature can provide us with answers to questions. This activity invites you to call on your natural surroundings to help you answer a question that you are carrying. Just like calling a friend (or texting, I suppose!), nature has a way of providing us with solutions to our problems in the strangest of ways.

Find a space to walk outdoors, and consider a question or dilemma you have been working on in your mind that hasn't resolved yet. You don't need to tell anyone what the issue is. You can just keep it in your mind as you go for a walk for the next 10 minutes. Pay attention to what is going on around you during the walk. What is nature telling you?

At the end of the walk, reflect on what you experienced. How does the experience that nature provided fit with the question you were thinking about on your walk? Were there clues that nature provided you with as you walked around? Don't overthink this. Use the following space to write the first thing that comes to your mind.

_____

_____

_____

_____

_____

_____

_____

_____

Adapted from McGeeney (2016)

Be a Good Neighbor

It has been said that nature is a colony of multiple nations that must learn to live together. There are different languages, cultures, and customs. Part of being a good neighbor is getting to know your own community. In this exercise, you will explore your neighborhood and look to see who (or what) cohabitates with you and your family. Is it a den of red foxes? A flock of geese? A nursery of raccoons? Or do you have deer that drink from a local creek? Who lives in your neighborhood, right next door? Go outside and take a walk around your neighborhood. Look for the creatures around you and answer the questions below to describe what you find.

Who are the neighborhood creatures that live in your community?

_____

_____

_____

Where do they live?

_____

_____

_____

What do they eat?

_____

_____

_____

Who are their best friends?

_____

_____

_____

Who are their enemies?

_____

_____

_____

Mini-Beast's Life

Sometimes, it seems that we are the only species that exists in the world. Yet we are surrounded by (and live among) many creatures—big and small. Being aware of the interrelatedness of living things is one way to promote empathy and altruism among children. In this activity, children are invited to explore the meadows and fields to discover that they are not the only creatures on this earth. They are among mini-beasts.

Preparation

- Sweep nets to catch the insects without harming them. You can use an old pillowcase or old nylons stretched out over a rounded coat hanger.
- Clear containers with lids to view the insects
- Magnifying glasses

Instructions

1. On a warm, sunny day, gather the children outside in a meadow or green space with long grass.

2. Use the sweep net to catch various creatures living in the grass.

3. Place one creature in each container, and pass it around for the group to look at.

4. Have children use a magnifying glass to look more carefully at each creature. Look at its color, shape, texture, and size. Be sure to take care of the creature so it does not get too hot or thirsty.

5. When everyone has had a chance to look at and discuss the creatures, return them to the long grass so that they may resume their happy, hoppy lives.

6. Encourage children to watch the creatures disappear back into their elements and imagine what it would be like to live life as a mini-beast.

Adapted from McGeeney (2016)

Group Fun:
Buried in Autumn Leaves

There is something beautiful about sitting quietly in nature. Many people understand the beauty of watching a sunrise or sunset, or sitting by the wide ocean. However, the quiet of nestling in a pile of leaves can also provide a moment of reflection and observation about the natural world around us. In addition, the swaddle of leaves can be both comforting and quieting. In this group activity, children will participate in the experience of being cared for by another. In particular, they will connect to the leaves with the quiet presence of a friend nearby.

Preparation
- A place outdoors with some wooded area and lots of leaves
- Comfortable clothes
- Whistle
- Small blanket or piece of tarp (optional)

Instructions
1. Have everyone in the group gather a big pile of leaves and form the leaves in the shape of a large rectangle.
2. Once the pile of leaves has been formed, ask the group to gather in silence around the rectangle and spend some time walking around the leaves with their bare feet.
3. After some time has passed (don't rush it!), have the children re-scatter the leaves around the ground with their feet.
4. Ask each child to choose a partner they feel comfortable with, and have each pair go off on their own and take turns burying each other in the leaves. Instruct children that there is no talking throughout the exercise and that they should leave their partner's face and eyes uncovered.
5. If children are unsure about laying on the leaves, they can lay on a blanket or tarp if they would prefer.
6. After the first child is buried with leaves, the burier sits quietly nearby while their partner enjoys the experience. The pairs swap turns when the group leader blows a whistle.
7. Don't rush the exercise. Simply encourage children to sit in silence with nature and a friend.
8. After each child in the dyad has completed the exercise, regather the group and ask some reflection questions. What did it feel like to be nestled in the pile of leaves? What was it like to lay quietly? What was it like to have a friend sit quietly by their side?

Adapted from McGeeney (2016)

chapter
NINE

Creating Inclusive Green Spaces and Activities

> *"When a flower doesn't bloom, you fix the environment in which it grows, not the flower."*
>
> — Alexander den Heijer

Concrete buildings with windowless walls and fluorescent lighting describe the clinical and learning environments endured by many children (and adults). Hard landscapes are abundant while green space is sparse, and the scholarly and scheduled demands of children leave little (if any) time for unplanned outdoor activities. Children spend less than an hour a week in unstructured outdoor play, whereas they spend an average of 44 hours a week on electrical devices. Additionally, 47 million Americans live in housing that prohibits children from playing outside! This includes rules against playing in treehouses, climbing trees, riding skateboards, shooting hoops, or even playing with sidewalk chalk (Souter-Brown, 2015).

However, the physical, mental, emotional, and spiritual benefits of engaging in green space cannot be understated (Arvay, 2018; Bailey, Howells, & Glibo, 2018; Combs, Hoag, Javorski, & Roberts, 2016; Guo, 2015). As we have learned, children become overwhelmed by the harsh stimuli of artificial lighting and hardscapes, which contribute to an array of behavioral issues, including difficulties with concentration, restlessness, and aggression. **Children need to unplug and engage in nondirective play in sensory-rich settings to build confidence, improve concentration, increase problem solving, and promote a calm and alert state.**

Not everyone is able to work in a natural setting, which is when we bring the outdoors indoors. Research has found that integrating green spaces into urban settings has numerous therapeutic benefits among children, including reduced aggression (Younan et al., 2016), increased attention and focus (Taylor & Kuo, 2011), and an increase in overall emotional well-being (Flouri, Midouhas, & Joshi, 2014). Therefore, creating green space for children is both therapeutic and necessary to counter the effects of our fast-paced, digitally-driven society and raise a generation of healthier and happier children. In this chapter, I'll discuss how you can bring the natural elements into your workplace, even in a windowless, concrete classroom or office.

TYPES OF GREEN SPACES

Nature-informed spaces offer reflective and calming areas that inspire imagination and improve emotional regulation. If you are fortunate enough to have some outdoor space, here are some tips for creating a variety of therapeutic spaces.

Children's Gardens

Creating gardens with children in mind will include opportunities to engage in whole-body and whole-brain experiences. Here are a few ideas:

- Create a space for sand and water play. For example, repurpose an old rowboat and fill it with sand. Children will spend hours simply moving water to sand and creating narratives around mythical creatures and magical structures molded by the sand and water. Include nature bins filled with shells, rocks, sea glass, sticks, feathers, and other small, natural elements to offer additional tools for imaginative play.

- Include climbing areas for crawling over and under things. Some schools are even creating climbing walls for children. Open fields can be enhanced by including play caves, tents, or tepees through which children crawl. You may want to include a small bridge or locate areas where there may be trees or fallen logs to climb over and around. Allow for walking paths and incorporate crawl options, such as tunnels or tubes. If you have a slight slope, you can craft a space for rolling or sliding. Areas that encourage navigating the terrain promote problem solving and confidence as children master the elements.

- Create discovery zones, such as bog gardens and herb patches. Perhaps there is a forest area or space around a lake or pond that can be sectioned off just for children to roam and explore. Keep discovery tools, such as sweep nets, garden gloves, clear containers, and magnifying glasses in an accessible location so that children can use them in their explorations. Allowing children to freely explore green space promotes interaction between the children and environment in a way that encourages connection and empathy.

- Develop an open-air theater where children can perform. Create a space that encourages children to build and play natural instruments. For example, children might choose to make drums using sticks and rocks, or bamboo flutes and gourd maracas. You may want to offer more traditional instruments as well and encourage musical expression among the open forum. Additionally, keep a box of props accessible for children to author their own screenplays in the open-air theater. The use of props in this open-air forum promotes creative expression and healthy interaction with the outdoor setting.

- Use outdoor space for art projects. An easy way to encourage children to engage in natural settings is to take art projects to the outdoors. The "Nature Staining" activity (Chapter 5)—in which children use the stain from berries and bark to draw or paint—is a great project for outdoor spaces. Additionally, sand collages, nature mandalas, and guerilla rocks are easy to set up and execute in an outdoor art space. Outdoor art spaces encourage creative expression while introducing children to the beauty and wonder in the natural world.

Sensory Garden

Sensory gardens capitalize on color, sound, fragrance, texture, and taste. Providing a variety of plants and natural stations will encourage children to engage all of their senses. In addition to colorful and fragrant plants and flowers, sensory gardens can include desertscapes and water gardens. Rock gardens also invite sensory engagement, and adding a rock balance station can provide an intentionally mindful focus to the garden.

Healing Garden

Healing gardens are intentionally crafted to create comfort and peaceful experiences. This type of garden is conducive to pediatric hospitals and rehabilitation centers. Fragrant flowers, gentle waterfalls, and plants that attract birds and butterflies provide soothing sights and sounds for children and their families. Adding a mandala or labyrinth to the garden can make it a place for reflection.

Teenage Den in the Woods

The desire to fit in and find a sense of belonging is the signature essence of the teen years, and teens look for their own special hangouts as they navigate the coming-of-age process. However, in current society, social media has provided a venue that has replaced soda shops, roller rinks, and burger joints of years gone by. What better way to encourage engaging with nature than to design a cozy outdoor den just for teens. Use benches and stumps for sitting areas, and hammocks for them to hang out on.

Barrel Ponds and Gardens

Empty barrels can be repurposed to provide containers for water and a variety of natural resources. These are easy to make and sustain. Use barrel halves filled with water, plants, sand, and rocks. Barrel gardens are contained and can be created in small spaces that provide children with nature-informed sensory stimuli.

Edible Garden

Edible gardens are fun to grow and even more fun to use for aromatherapy, as well as foraging feasts. You can include a variety of herbs and flowers for steeping, smelling, and tasting. An edible garden introduces children to the many properties of plants, in addition to the interdependence between plants and people, as they create snacks from the flowers and herbs.

Nature Collaboration

Even if you do not have outdoor green space in your immediate vicinity, there are many different ways to collaborate with existing green resources in the community. For example, you can schedule visits to a local nature center, botanical garden, butterfly conservatory, or zoo, and have children subsequently discuss the experience. If you are a clinician, you can locate a labyrinth near you (https://labyrinthlocator.com) and invite children and their caregivers to walk the space prior to a session with you, or you can have them do so afterward as a means of grounding and processing what was discussed in session. You can also connect with a forest guide (https://www.natureandforesttherapy.org/membership/member-directory#!directory/map/ord=lnm) in your area and have children experience a mindful forest guided walk. These forest walks can help children cultivate an attitude of mindful reflection, challenge their physical comfort, and connect with biodiversity in an intentional way.

GREEN SPACES FOR ALL: MAKING SURE YOUR SPACE IS INCLUSIVE

Helen Keller once observed that people were surprised that she could enjoy nature. It was really they, she said, who were blind, "for they have no idea how fair the flower is to the touch, nor do they appreciate its fragrance, which is the soul of the flower." Although every child can enjoy green space, it is important to consider inclusion when designing the space. Is the space conducive for wheelchairs or other apparatuses? How do children with visual or hearing impairment navigate the space? The following are some factors to consider to help make your space more inclusive:

- Create raised garden beds to accommodate children in wheelchairs.
- Provide wide pathways so children with walkers and wheelchairs can easily turn around.

- Create the green space on level ground to prevent possible falls.
- Store child-informed gardening tools near the gardens in the same easily accessible location.
- For children who are not sighted, place a small radio (and play nature sounds or soothing music) at the same point of the garden to orient the child to the garden design. In this way, the child can familiarize him- or herself with the garden and navigate it with little assistance.
- Include a watering pitcher with drip valve for children who are blind or partially sighted.

In addition to sensory inclusion, cultural gardens offer a gardening experience inclusive of a variety of terrain. Using plants indigenous to specific cultural areas, cultural gardens expose children to different plants and landscapes found in a variety of countries and locations. For example, I spent part of my childhood in the tropics of the Philippine Islands. Luscious fruits and fragrant flowers surrounded my home, school, and neighborhood. I still become nostalgic when I see the white and yellow frangipani flowers. Additionally, creating a culture garden can be a great alternative or addition to routine multicultural festivals.

BRINGING NATURE INDOORS

If you find yourself working with children behind windowless concrete, do not despair.

There are numerous ways to bring nature indoors to your practice as well. A hybrid version may include an intentionally-crafted entrance to your setting. For example, you can create a nature scape right outside your door by including potted plants, a water fountain, or a rock garden in your waiting area. You may also want to include a variety of bird feeders or butterfly plants in the outside entrance to your environment.

Another way to bring nature indoors is to have your workspace reflect the seasonal changes. Bring in natural elements to your office that correspond with the particular time of year, such as sea glass and seashells for the summer and colored leaves in the fall. I like to keep a variety of essential oils in my desk and rotate seasonal plants into my office. For example, I may choose a poinsettia in the winter, a small mum in the autumn, rosemary or mint in the summer, and daffodils and clover in the springtime.

Bringing nature into your space is only limited by your imagination. I decided a long time ago that I wanted to work in a setting that reminded me of a beach cottage, and I specifically chose my furniture, colors, and accents with this intention. Wicker sofas and chairs donned with teal and blue, bookshelves hosting driftwood, and sea glass and shells mingled among the books. An electric fireplace and a soft throw offer cozy warmth during the winter months. Creating a nature-informed space is not only inviting to the children with whom you work, but it provides you with a much-needed haven.

Nature-Informed Technology

We live in a technological society where children as young as two years old are plugged into their devices. Although the recommended dose of tablet time is 60 minutes a day, most of us well exceed this in our use of computers, televisions, and telephones. While it is true that we need to balance our digital time with time spent outdoors in nature, the use of nature-informed technology can be of therapeutic benefit when outside options are limited. For example, research has found that live webcams of nature can reduce stress, promote emotion regulation, and increase productivity (Kahn, Severson, & Ruckert, 2009). Moreover, these therapeutic effects are specific to scenes that depict nature, as these same effects are not observed with videos that portray urban environments.

Therefore, adding a nature-informed tablet in your office with changing scenes of outdoor land and seascapes may be therapeutic for you and the children you see. Additionally, you can substitute nature sounds—such as ocean waves, soft rainfall, or leaves rustling in the wind—in lieu of a music playlist. You can also incorporate the use of nature-based video games, such as Walden, which encourage interaction between the child and the virtual forest and natural setting. Although engaging with the outdoors is certainly the more preferable option, nature-informed technology is better than no nature at all.

COST-EFFECTIVE FUNDING: MAKING YOUR GREEN SPACE A REALITY

Accessing the resources needed to create green space can feel daunting, as most budgets are already shoestring tight. However, here are a few creative ways to actualize your nature-informed dreams:

- **Grant funding:** Look for funding through not only environmental groups, but through products as well. For example, Scotts Miracle-Gro held an initiative to help fund 1,000 community gardens and green spaces between 2011 and 2018 (their 150th anniversary).
- **Crowdfunding:** Consider creating a funding website for your project. Social media has become a great venue to solicit donations for your green space. Additionally, parent-teacher groups and local child-centric interest groups may contribute to the cause.
- **Guerilla gardening:** This project costs little to promote green space. Just make and/ or purchase seed bombs or seed packets, and distribute them to the community with the instructions to "plant a garden in the most unlikely of places."

THE POWER OF PLANTS: A CASE STUDY

The power of bringing nature indoors is exemplified through the efforts of Stephen Ritz, a high school teacher in the Bronx who worked at a school plagued by abysmal attendance and graduation rates. Through the use of a "green curriculum," Ritz transformed the lives of his students by cultivating an environment of enthusiasm and academic excellence. In particular, Ritz incorporated tower garden technology into his classroom, which is a self-sustaining indoor ecosystem, and created a comprehensive curriculum around the system. Students learned math and science while tilling dirt, planting seeds, and harvesting the produce. The students produced so much that they brought the surplus of fresh vegetables home to their families. Nutrition and cooking were added to the curriculum, and students began creating a garden to table experience.

Not only did his students' attendance improve, but so did their test scores. In addition, his students learned skills that translated to jobs when they graduated. Eventually, Ritz's movement grew—with the production of these tower gardens spanning across the city—and Ritz founded the Green Bronx Machine, which now hosts produce and food for an entire community. This poor urban community experienced hope of a different life for its children, all because of a creative and motivated high school teacher—and a tower garden system. In the words of Stephen Ritz, "When we teach children about nature, we teach them to nurture, and when we teach children to nurture, we as a society collectively embrace our better nature" (2017, p. 260).

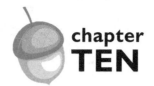

chapter
TEN

Where Do We Go from Here? Resources for Nature-Based Mindfulness Practices

"Do not go where the path may lead, go instead where there is no path and leave a trail."

— Ralph Waldo Emerson

I have had the opportunity over the past few years to present lectures and workshops on the benefits of mindfulness and nature-informed tools to educators and clinicians all over the country. As most scholars discover, I, too, have taken away so much more from my participants who have attended my workshops and lectures. One of the things I have learned is that the desire to reconnect to nature is worldwide and spans disciplines. Practitioners from all fields are studying and applying the foundational benefits of nature's wisdom in profound ways. Inspired, where do we go from here?

ECOTHERAPY AND ECOPSYCHOLOGY PROGRAMS

Ecotherapy, or ecopsychology, refers to the integration of psychotherapy or psychology and nature. It can include, but is not limited to, horticulture therapy (healing through gardening), animal-assisted therapy (healing through therapeutic interactions with animals), wilderness therapy (therapeutic integration of wilderness immersions), and nature-informed therapy (therapeutic integration of natural elements with traditional therapeutic approaches). Both ecotherapy and ecopsychology programs emphasize the interrelatedness between psychology and the human-nature connection. The underlying premise is that humanity was formed within the natural setting, and it is detachment from our natural roots that has resulted in dis-ease. Therefore, eco-therapeutic approaches promote the reconnection of individuals to the earth and its elements, and advocate for sustainable and restorative ecological practices.

Ecotherapy and ecopsychology graduate programs and certifications are available all over the world, including 28 programs in the United States. Graduate programs include those at the master's and doctoral level, which involve didactic and nature immersion components. Training involves both academics and research to address the therapeutic features of integrating nature in a clinical practice, assessment and treatment planning, modifications for diverse populations, and ethical considerations. Programs do not typically culminate in license eligibility for counselors, social workers, or other mental health practitioners, and many programs require or recommend current licensure to enroll. Certifications range from exclusively online to hybrid formats, as well as immersion-only intensive programs that can be completed in one week to several months with supervision included. Here is a link to get you started: http://www.apadivisions.org/division-34/about/resources/graduate-programs.aspx.

THE ASSOCIATION OF NATURE AND FOREST THERAPY

The Association of Nature and Forest Therapy is a global leader in promoting the development and practice of forest therapy. As discussed in Chapter 2, forest therapy or forest bathing is the practice of spending time in the forest to improve health and overall wellness. A certified forest therapy guide facilitates the forest walk and invites participants to connect intentionally to the natural elements they discover on the walk. To achieve certification as a forest guide, individuals must complete a week of intensive training, followed by six months of supervision and application. Immersions and certifications are offered all over the world. If you are interested, you can learn more at: http://www.natureandforesttherapy.org.

TIMBERNOOK

TimberNook, an outdoor nature program for children, was developed by occupational therapist Angela Hanscom. TimberNook is based on the assumption that all children flourish when given the time and space to play in sensory-rich, experiential learning environments that challenge the mind, body, and the senses through meaningful outdoor play opportunities. Hanscom provides weeklong intensive trainings that consists of five days of hands-on learning at TimberNook's 12-acre wooded headquarters in Barrington, New Hampshire, and New Zealand, followed by a three-day onsite training at your program launch. Additionally, TimberNook provides a business model that promotes the successful launching and sustainability of new programs. For more information, visit: http://www.timbernook.com.

NATIONAL ORGANIZATIONS

Children & Nature Network

The Children & Nature Network is a U.S.-based program whose mission is to "increase equitable access to nature so that children—and natural places—can thrive. We do this by investing in leadership and communities through sharing evidence-based resources, scaling innovative solutions and driving policy change" (https://www.childrenandnature.org). The organization connects individuals with institutions to facilitate social change; provides training through webinars, leadership summits, and annual conferences; and supports research efforts with the goal of increasing access to nature. In addition, it promotes a variety of related community initiatives, such as Cities Connecting Children to Nature (which creates nature-rich cities and improved nature access for low-income communities), Green Schoolyards (which transforms schoolyards into green spaces for children), and Natural Families (which serves over 35,000 families and encourages engaging in frequent active outdoor time together).

Center for Ecopsychology

The Center for Ecopsychology was founded in August 2000 to meet the growing demand for both professional trainings and academic courses in ecopsychology. The center offers both noncredit professional trainings and for-credit academic courses, including a 16-credit certificate program in ecopsychology. The certificate in ecopsychology is available either as an on-campus or an online program: https://www.ecopsychology.org/.

Every Kid in the Park

Every Kid in the Park is a national incentive to assure that fourth graders and their families can access wildlife resources and history free of charge through partnerships with national organizations, parks, and historic sites: https://www.everykidinapark.gov/.

Geocaching

Geocaching has been described as "a real-world, outdoor treasure hunting game using GPS-enabled devices." Navigating to a specific set of GPS coordinates, children search for the geocache (container) hidden at that location. The geocaching community manages the containers so all you need to get started is a GPS device or a GPS-enabled mobile phone. Visit their website for more information: https://www.geocaching.com/play.

Kids4Trees

Kids4Trees works with national and local forests and community organizations to connect kids with nature. Through free environmental education, they provide a variety of programs including tree planting and other events for 6- to 12-year-old children: http://www.kids4trees.org/.

National Environmental Education Foundation's Children and Nature Initiative

This organization educates healthcare providers working with children about the benefits of outdoor activities for children. It also connects providers with local nature organizations to refer families to easily accessible outdoor areas: https://www.neefusa.org/.

PBS Kids Plum Landing

PBS Kids is a project from WGBH Boston that introduces families and educators to easy and fun activities that encourage kids to get outside and connect to nature. You can access their games, activities, and videos at their site: https://pbskids.org/plumlanding/educators/index.html.

The National Wildlife Federation

The National Wildlife Federation is a national organization whose mission is to protect natural resources, restore ecosystems, and educate and connect individuals and communities to wildlife: https://www.nwf.org/About-Us/Our-Mission.

Let's G.O.! (Get Outside)

Let's G.O.! is an initiative of the Children & Nature Network that encourages people of all ages to get outside and spend time in nature. Families, teachers, students, mentors, grandparents, and friends—especially children and youth—are urged to participate: https://www.childrenandnature.org/initiatives/letsgo/.

LOCAL GROUPS

Ancestral Knowledge (Maryland)

Ancestral Knowledge is a nonprofit organization that provides workshops and retreats for children, families, and homeschoolers on topics such as seasonal foraging, primitive skills building, and the wildcrafting of pens, inks, and crayons: https://www.ancestralknowledge.org.

Delaware Nature Society (Delaware)

The Delaware Nature Society promotes the discovery of nature for all ages through camps, educational programs, and fun events. Check it out at https://www.delawarenaturesociety.org/activities/education/.

Desert Botanical Garden (Arizona)

The Desert Botanical Garden encourages children to connect with nature by providing a variety of environmental educational and experiential programs, ranging from early childhood to adolescence: https://www.dbg.org/learn/children-families-educators/.

Earthshine Nature Program (Carolinas)

Earthshine Nature Program educates children about wildlife and nature conservation, nature awareness, and renewable energy. The program has a particular specialty in reptile rescue: http://earthshinenature.com/.

Earth Walk (Vermont)

Earth Walk is a nonprofit organization in Vermont that aspires to reconnect children and families to their natural heritage through retreats and programs: https://www.earthwalkvermont.org/.

Houston Arboretum and Nature Center (Texas)

Children between the ages of 18 months and 12 years will find developmentally-appropriate adventures in natural settings as they learn to navigate the terrain through a variety of hands-on activities: https://houstonarboretum.org/childrens-programs/.

Junior Ranger Program (North Carolina)

Through the Junior Ranger Program, children gain an appreciation of North Carolina's cultural and natural heritage and learn about careers in natural resources: https://www.ncparks.gov/junior-rangers.

Magnolia Nature School (Alabama)

Magnolia Nature School is Alabama's first outdoor preschool and camp where children between the ages of three and six can explore farms, forests, and streams: https://campmcdowell.com/educational-programs/magnolia-nature-school.

North Carolina Botanical Garden (North Carolina)

The Botanical Garden hosts a variety of family-friendly activities that include the exploration of flora and fauna found in the Wonder Garden: http://ncbg.unc.edu/youth-family/.

NOVA Parks (Virginia)

Through a variety of programs (guided nature walks), activities (hikes), and events (night explorations and stream and pond studies), children learn about plants and animals in a safe and fun way: https://www.novaparks.com/things-to-do/naturalists.

Ohio Nature Education (Ohio)

Ohio Nature Education provides a variety of fun and interesting programs that introduce children to animals, bird nests, and other natural elements: https://www.ohionature.org/programs.

Owl's Hill Nature Sanctuary (Tennessee)

Owl's Hill provides environmental education programs for children and adults. Children experience fun programs that include guided hiking through a variety of habitats. They can visit with the owls, learn about them, and discover why they call Owl's Hill home: http://www.owlshill.org.

Penn State Better Kid Care (Pennsylvania)

Penn State Better Kid Care provides research-based education to early learning and school-aged professionals about the benefits of connecting children with nature. http://www.betterkidcare.psu.edu.

Santa Cruz Kids in Nature Program (California)

This is an outdoor-based nature club for children aged 5–10. Through a multitude of afterschool activities, the program fosters creativity, confidence, communication skills, community, ecological stewardship, and curiosity in children: https://www.kidsinnaturesc.com/.

Stage Nature Center (Michigan)

Stage Nature Center provides developmentally-appropriate nature programs to children of all ages and stages. Beginning with "Knee-high Naturalists" through "Little Acorns," children discover the secrets found in natural settings: https://troynaturesociety.org/programs/programs_children/.

Wesselman Nature Society (Indiana)

Wesselman Nature Society connects children to nature through nature preschools and a variety of outdoor programs that will ignite the innate naturalist in any child: https://www.wesselmanwoods.com/activities-programs/programs-for-kids/.

CONCLUSION

Nature is an accessible and cost-effective co-therapist that inspires awe and wonder. It provides children with a whole-body, whole-brain, multisensory, complex experience that promotes the development of cognitive, physical, and emotional growth. As clinicians, we can bring nature's wisdom into our practices and help children reestablish a holistic sense of wellness and agency in their lives. We can promote a therapeutic connection to natural elements. Atkins and Snyder (2018) capture this essence in the following parable:

An elder once asked a young person he was working with, "Are you a medicine woman?" She hesitated, afraid of making too much of herself. He challenged her saying, "This is not about you. The ancestors and the future beings are waiting for you to show up and claim your inheritance." This is our call and our response/ability as nature-based expressive artists—to claim and use the medicine of the arts and the Earth in the service of all life. (Atkins & Snyder, 2018, p. 134)

Join the conversation and see what unfolds for you and your practice.

References

For your convenience, purchasers can download and print worksheets and handouts from www.pesi.com/NatureTools

Abreu, T., & Figueiredo, A. (2015). Paws for help—Animal-assisted therapy. *European Psychiatry, 30,* 1651.

Ahn, R. R., Miller, L. J., Milberger, S., & McIntosh, D. N. (2004). Prevalence of parents' perceptions of sensory processing disorders among kindergarten children. *American Journal of Occupational Therapy, 58,* 287–302.

Andrews, C. R., & Marotta, S. A. (2005). Spirituality and coping among grieving children: A preliminary study. *Counseling and Values, 50*(1), 38–50.

Arvay, C. G. (2018). *The healing code of nature: Discovering the new science of eco-psychomatics.* Boulder, CO: Sounds True Publishing.

Atkins, S., & Snyder, M. (2018). *Nature-based expressive arts therapy: Integrating the expressive arts and ecotherapy.* London, UK: Jessica Kingsley Publisher.

Baer, J. (2016). Creativity doesn't develop in a vacuum. *New Directions for Child and Adolescent Development, 151,* 9–20.

Baer, J., & Kaufman, J. C. (2012). *Being creative inside and outside the classroom.* Rotterdam, The Netherlands: Sense Publishers.

Bailey, R. P., Howells, K., & Glibo, I. (2018). Physical activity and mental health of school-aged children and adolescents: A rapid review. *International Journal of Physical Education, 55*(1), 2–15.

Banning, W., & Sullivan, G. (2011). *Lens on outdoor learning.* St. Paul, MN: Redleaf Press.

Beetz, A. M. (2017). Theories and possible processes of action in animal-assisted interventions. *Applied Developmental Science, 21*(2), 139–149.

Beghetto, R. A. (2013). *Killing ideas softly? The promise and perils of creativity in the classroom.* Charlotte, NC: Information Age Publishing.

Berger, R. (2016). Renewed by nature: Nature therapy as a framework to help people deal with crises, trauma and loss. In M. Jordan and J. Hinds (Eds.), *Ecotherapy: Theory, research and practice* (pp. 177–186). London, UK: Palgrave.

Berger, R., & Lahad, M. (2013). *The healing forest in post-crisis work with children: A nature therapy and expressive arts program for groups.* London, UK: Jessica Kingsley Publishers.

Berger, R., & McLeod, J. (2006). Incorporating nature into therapy: A framework for practice. *Journal of Systemic Therapies, 25*(2), 80–94.

Buzzel, L. & Chalquist, C. (Eds.). (2009). *Ecotherapy: Healing with nature in mind.* Berkeley, CA: Counterpoint Publishing.

Campbell, D. (2011, May 21). Children growing weaker as computers replace outdoor activities. *The Guardian.* Retrieved from https://www.theguardian.com/society/2011/may/21/children-weaker-computers-replace-activity

Campbell, J. (1991). *The power of myth.* New York, NY: First Anchor Books.

Carr, N. (2011). *The shallows: What the internet is doing to our brains.* New York, NY: W. W. Norton.

Chown, A. (2018). *A practical guide to play therapy in the outdoors: Working in nature.* New York, NY: Routledge.

Combs, K., Hoag, M., Javorski, S., & Roberts, S. (2016). Adolescent self-assessment of an outdoor behavioral health program: Longitudinal outcomes and trajectories of change. *Journal of Child and Family Studies, 25*(11), 3322–3330.

Dawson, J. (2016). Empathy through animals: Generating evidence-based outcomes for empathy development. *Juvenile and Family Court Journal, 67*(4), 43–54.

Delaney, T. (2008). *The sensory processing disorder answer book: Practical answers to the top 250 questions parents ask.* Naperville, IL: Sourcebooks.

DiCiacco, J. A. (2008). *The colors of grief: Understanding a child's journey through loss from birth to adulthood.* London, UK: Jessica Kingsley Publishers.

Dietz, W. H. (2015). The health effects of green space: Then and now. *International Journal of Obesity, 39,* 1329.

Dunlop, K., & Tsantefski, M. (2017). A space of safety: Children's experience of equine-assisted group therapy. *Child and Family Social Work, 23*(1), 16–24.

Faramarzi, S., Rad, S. A., & Abedi, A. (2016). Effect of sensory integration training on executive functions of children with attention deficit hyperactivity disorder. *Neuropsychiatry & Neuropsychology, 11*(1), 1–5.

Farmer, P. (2014). Ecotherapy for mental health. *Journal of Holistic Healthcare, 11*(1), 18–21.

Felitti, V. J., Anda, R. F., Nordenberg, D., Williamson, D. F., Spitz, A. M., Edwards, V., & Marks, J. S. (1998). Relationship of childhood abuse and household dysfunction to many of the leading causes of death in adults: The Adverse Childhood Experiences (ACE) Study. *American Journal of Preventive Medicine, 14*(4), 245–258.

Fisher, A. V., Godwin, K. E., & Seltman, H. (2014). Visual environment attention allocation, and learning in young children: When too much of a good thing may be bad. *Psychological Science, 25*(7), 1362–1370.

Fisher, C. (2016, November 17). The counseling connoisseur: Mini-mindfulness moments. *Counseling Today Online.* Retrieved from https://ct.counseling.org/2016/11/counseling-connoisseur-mini-mindfulness-moments/

Fisher, C. (2017, November 27). The counseling connoisseur: Eco-culture: Clinical application of nature-informed therapy. *Counseling Today Online.* Retrieved from https://ct.counseling.org/2017/11/the-counseling-connoisseur-eco-culture-clinical-application-of-nature-informed-therapy/

Flouri, E., Midouhas, E., & Joshi, H. (2014). The role of urban neighbourhood green space in children's emotional and behavioural resilience. *Journal of Environmental Psychology, 40,* 179–186.

Goodman-Scott, E., & Lambert, S. F. (2015). Professional counseling for children with sensory processing disorder. *The Professional Counselor, 5*(2), 273–292

Gray, D. P. (2012). As children's freedom has declined, so has their creativity. *Psychology Today.* Retrieved from https://www.psychologytoday.com/us/blog/freedom-learn/201209/children-s-freedom-has-declined-so-has-their-creativity

Green, A., & Corson, D. (2009). *A guide to implementing sensory strategies in the classroom setting.* Stuart, FL: Therapy Interventions.

Growth Point. (1999). Your future starts here: Practitioners determine the way ahead. *Growth Point, 79,* 4–5.

Guo, T. (2015). Recreation of agricultural landscape for children with nature-deficit disorder. *Journal of Landscape Research, 7*(5), 14–16.

Hales, C. M., Carroll, M. D., Fryar, C. D., & Ogden, C. L. (2017). Prevalence of obesity among adults and youth: United States, 2015–2016. *NCHS Data Brief No. 288,* 1–8.

Hanh, T. N. (2011). *Planting seeds: Practicing mindfulness with children.* Berkley, CA: Parallax Press.

Hanh, T. N. (2012). *A handful of quiet: Happiness in four pebbles.* Berkeley, CA: Plum Blossom Books.

Hanscom, A. (2016). *Balanced and barefoot.* Oakland, CA: Harbinger Publishing.

Hart, T. (2003). *The secret spiritual world of children: The breakthrough discovery that profoundly alters our conventional view of children's mystical experiences.* Novato, CA: New World Library.

Hughes, K., Bellis, M. A., Hardcastle, K. A., Sethi, D., Butchart, A., Mikton, C., … & Dunne, M. P. (2017). The effect of multiple adverse childhood experiences on health: A systematic review and meta-analysis. *The Lancet Public Health, 2*(8), e356–e366.

Hyde, B. (2008). *Children and spirituality: Searching for meaning and connectedness.* Philadelphia, PA: Jessica Kingsley Publishers.

Jordan, M. (2014). Moving beyond counselling and psychotherapy as it currently is—Taking therapy outside. *European Journal of Psychotherapy & Counselling, 16*(4), 361–375.

Jordan, M. (2015). *Nature and therapy: Understanding counselling and psychotherapy in outdoor space.* London, UK: Routledge Publishing.

Kabat-Zinn, J. (2003). Mindfulness-based interventions in context: Past, present, and future. *Clinical Psychology: Science and Practice, 10,* 144–156.

Kabat-Zinn, J. (2013). *Full catastrophe living: Using the wisdom of your body and mind to address stress, pain and illness.* New York, NY: Random House.

Kahn, P. H., Severson, R. L., & Ruckert, J. H. (2009). The human relation with nature and technological nature. *Current Directions in Psychological Science, 18*(1), 37–42.

Kahn, P., & Kellert, S. (2002). *Children and nature: Psychological, sociocultural, and evolutionary investigations.* Cambridge, MA: MIT Press.

Kann, L., Kinchen, S., Shanklin, S. L., Flint, K. H., Hawkins, J., Harris, W. A. … Zara, S. (2014). Youth risk behavior surveillance—United States, 2013. *Morbidity and Mortality Weekly Report Surveillance Summaries, 63*(4), 1–18.

Kellert, S. (2002). *Children and nature: Psychological, sociocultural, and evolutionary investigations.* Cambridge, MA: MIT Press.

Kim, K. H. (2011). The creativity crisis: The decrease in creative thinking scores on the Torrance Tests of Creative Thinking. *Creativity Research Journal, 23*(4), 285–295.

Koenig, K., Huecker, G., & Kinnealey, M. (2005, May). *Comparative outcomes of children with ADHD: Treatment versus delayed treatment control condition.* Paper presented at the American Occupational Therapy Association Annual Conference and Exposition, Long Beach, California.

Kosfeld, M., Heinrichs, M., Zak, P. J., Fischbacher, U., & Fehr, E. (2005). Oxytocin increases trust in humans. *Nature, 435*(7042), 673.

Lahad, M. (2006). *Fantastic reality.* Haifa, Israel: Nord Publishing.

Lahad, M., Shacham, M., & Ayalon, O. (2013). *The "BASIC Ph" model of coping and resiliency: Theory, research and cross-cultural application.* London, UK: Jessica Kingsley Publishers.

Li, Q. (2018). *Forest bathing: How trees can help you find health and happiness.* New York, NY: Random House.

Louv, R. (2008). *The last child in the woods: Saving our children from nature-deficiency disorder.* Chapel Hill, NC: Algonquin Books.

Louv, R. (2012). *The nature principle: Reconnecting with life in a virtual age.* Chapel Hill, NC: Algonquin Books.

Louv, R. (2016). *Vitamin D: 500 ways to enrich the health & happiness of your family & community.* Chapel Hill, NC: Algonquin Books.

Mayer-Davis, E. J., Lawrence, J. M., Dabelea, D., Divers, J., Isom, S., Dolan, L., … Wagenknecht, L. (2017). Incidence trends of type 1 and type 2 diabetes among youths, 2002–2012. *New England Journal of Medicine, 376*(15), 1419–1429.

McGeeney, A. (2016). *With nature in mind: The ecotherapy manual for mental health professionals.* London, UK: Jessica Kingsley Publisher.

National Association for Mental Illness. (2018). *Mental health facts: Children & teens.* Retrieved from https://www.nami.org/NAMI/media/NAMI-Media/Infographics/Children-MH-Facts-NAMI.pdf

National Survey of Children's Health. (2011/12). *Data query from the Child and Adolescent Health Measurement Initiative.* Data Resource Center for Child and Adolescent Health. Retrieved from https://www.childhealthdata.org/browse/survey/results?q=2614&r=1

Natural Start Alliance. (2017, November 17). *Nature preschools and kindergartens at record numbers in the U.S.* Retrieved from https://naturalstart.org/bright-ideas/nature-preschools-and-kindergartens-record-numbers-us

Nover, A. G. (1985). Mother-infant interactive play: Theory and practical application. *Child and Adolescent Social Work Journal, 2*(1), 22–35.

Ober, C., Sinatra, S., & Zucker, M. (2014). *Earthing: The most important health discovery ever!* Laguna Beach, CA: Basic Health Publications.

O'Brien, M. E. R., Anderson, H., Kaukel, E., O'Byrne, K., Pawlicki, M., Von Pawel, J., & Reck, M. (2004). SRL172 (killed Mycobacterium vaccae) in addition to standard chemotherapy improves quality of life without affecting survival, in patients with advanced non-small-cell lung cancer: Phase III results. *Annals of Oncology, 15*(6), 906–914.

Ohio State University Center for Clinical and Translational Science. (2014, November 20). Scientists study effects of sunlight to reduce number of nearsighted kids. *ScienceDaily.* Retrieved from http://www.sciencedaily.com/releases/2014/11/141120112348.htm

Olmert, M. D. (2009). *Made for each other: The biology of the human-animal bond.* Cambridge, MA: DaCapo Press.

Pargament, K. (2011). *Spiritually integrated psychotherapy: Understanding and addressing the sacred.* New York, NY: Guilford Press.

Parker, K. J., Oztan, O., Libove, R. A., Sumiyoshi, R. D., Jackson, L. P., Karhson, D. S., … & Hardan, A. Y. (2017). Intranasal oxytocin treatment for social deficits and biomarkers of response in children with autism. *Proceedings of the National Academy of Sciences, 114*(30), 8119–8124.

Racette, S. B., Dill, T. C., White, M. L., Castillo, J. C., Uhrich, M. L., Inman, C. L. … Clark, B. R. (2015). Influence of physical education on moderate-to-vigorous physical activity of urban public school children in St. Louis, Missouri, 2011–2014. *Preventing Chronic Disease, 12*, 140458.

RB-Banks, Y., & Meyer, J. (2017). Childhood trauma in today's urban classroom: Moving beyond the therapist's office. *Educational Foundations, 30*(1–4), 63–75.

Ritz, S. (2017). *The power of a plant.* New York, NY: Rodale.

Russo, L. (2013). Play and creativity at the center of curriculum and assessment: A New York City school's journey to re-think curricular pedagogy. *Bordón, 65*(1), 131–146.

Siegel, D. J. (2012). *The developing mind: How relationships and the brain interact to shape who we are* (2nd ed.). New York, NY: Guilford Press.

Souter-Brown, G. (2014). *Landscape and urban design for health and well-being: Using healing, sensory and therapeutic gardens.* New York, NY: Routledge.

Sweeney, T. (2013). *Eco-art therapy*. London, UK: Jessica Kingsley Publishers.

Taylor, A. F., & Kuo, F. (2011). Could exposure to everyday green spaces help treat ADHD? Evidence from children's play settings. *Applied Psychology: Health and Well-Being, 3*(3), 281–303.

Tsantefski, M., Briggs, L., Griffiths, J., & Tidyman, A. (2017). An open trial of equine-assisted therapy for children exposed to problematic parental substance use. *Health & Social Care in the Community, 25*(3), 1247–1256.

van der Kolk, B. A. (2015). *The body keeps the score: Brain, mind, and body in the healing of trauma.* New York, NY: Penguin Books.

Visser, S. N., Danielson, M. L., Bitsko, R. H., Holbrook, J. R., Kogan, M. D., Ghandour, R. M., … Blumberg, S. J. (2014). Trends in the parent-report of healthcare provider diagnosed and medicated attention deficit hyperactive disorder: United States, 2003–2011. *Journal of American Academy of Child and Adolescent Psychiatry, 53*(1), 34–36.

Wilson, E. O. (2017). *The origins of creativity.* New York, NY: Liveright Publishing Corporation.

Worden, J. W. (2001). *Grief counseling and grief therapy: A handbook for the mental health professional* (3rd ed.). London, UK: Springer.

Younan, D., Tuvblad, C., Li, L., Wu, J., Lurmann, F., Franklin, M., & … Chen, J. (2016). Environmental determinants of aggression in adolescents: Role of urban neighborhood green space. *Journal of the American Academy of Child & Adolescent Psychiatry, 55*(7), 591–601.